Effective Group The
for Young Adults Affeⅽⅰeu
by Cancer

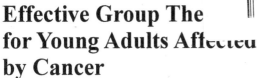

Outlining the unique psychosocial and development issues faced by young adults affected by cancer, this text draws on qualitative data from two pilot studies conducted in the United States to illustrate how the needs of this often-overlooked population can be effectively met via group therapy in clinical settings.

Drawing on 25 years of experience as a licensed clinical social worker supporting pediatric and young adult cancer patients and their families, Kurker focuses on the role of the clinician in structuring support group sessions. Chapters draw on patient perspectives to demonstrate effective application of interventions to help adolescents work through trauma associated with a diagnosis of cancer, treatment, recovery and the impacts on their development. Outcomes from these studies also include strategies for selecting support group participants, structuring group activities and securing funding.

Effective Group Therapies for Young Adults Affected by Cancer will be a valuable text for oncology social workers and clinicians involved in adolescent support services. In addition, researchers and postgraduate students with an interest in the fields of social work, psychology and adolescent development will find the book of interest.

Sarah F. Kurker, MSW, LICSW, is an Instructor in the Department of Social Work, Arizona State University, United States. She is also a practicing Clinical Social Worker and Oncology Teen and Young Adult Support Group Facilitator, Tucson, Arizona, United States.

Explorations in Mental Health

Frantz Fanon's Psychotherapeutic Approaches to Clinical Work
Practicing Internationally with Marginalized Communities
Edited by Lou Turner and Helen A. Neville

Deinstitutionalizing Art of the Nomadic Museum
Practicing and Theorizing Critical Art Therapy with Adolescents
Eva Marxen

Applications of a Psychospiritual Model in the Helping Professions
Principles of InnerView Guidance
Cedric Speyer and John Yaphe

Effective Group Therapies for Young Adults Affected by Cancer
Using Support Groups in Clinical Settings in the US
Sarah F. Kurker

Fostering Resilience Before, During, and After Experiences of Trauma
Insights to Inform Practice Across the Lifetime
Edited by Buuma Maisha, Stephanie Massicotte and Melanie Morin

For more information about this series, please visit www.routledge.com/ Explorations-in-Mental-Health/book-series/EXMH

Effective Group Therapies for Young Adults Affected by Cancer

Using Support Groups in Clinical Settings in the US

Sarah F. Kurker

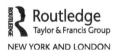
Routledge
Taylor & Francis Group

NEW YORK AND LONDON

First published 2021
by Routledge
52 Vanderbilt Avenue, New York, NY 10017

and by Routledge
2 Park Square, Milton Park, Abingdon, Oxon, OX14 4RN

*Routledge is an imprint of the Taylor & Francis Group,
an informa business*

Library of Congress Cataloging-in-Publication Data
A catalog record for this book has been requested

ISBN: 978-0-367-53381-6 (hbk)
ISBN: 978-0-367-53382-3 (pbk)
ISBN: 978-1-003-08170-8 (ebk)

Typeset in Times New Roman
by Apex CoVantage, LLC

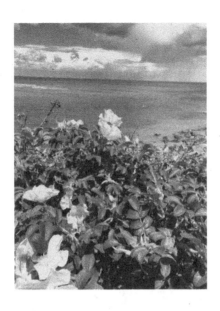

In memory of "Gabe."

Sure you can publish it but please don't use my full name!

A sincere thank you to every young adult who has shared your cancer experience with me. I feel honored of your trust. You have inspired me to become a better social worker.

A deep remembrance to each pediatric and adult patient I have known in my years as an oncology social worker. Always in my heart to be a grateful and appreciative.

For my children Emily and Evan who bring me happiness. May you follow your dreams and know I am here always. Thank you Kevin for supporting me.

For my parents Mickey and Frances Kurker for encouraging me to follow my dreams of becoming an oncology social worker.

To social workers at Massachusetts General Hospital and in Tucson, Arizona that I have had the privilege to work with.

To my Arizona State University Social Work Colleagues, thank you for your continued dedication to others.

A sincere thank you to Joanne Cacciatore for your time and support and teaching me so much by your research

For Elsbeth Wright (Routledge Taylor & Francis Editor—Education, Psychology & Mental Health Research), who believed in my vision of this book. Thank you for providing critical feedback that has allowed my dream of writing a book about young adults with cancer a reality.

Nature and movement: for keeping me in the moment of appreciation.

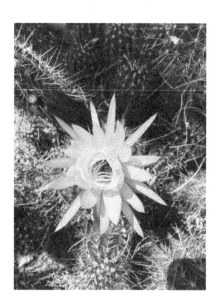

Contents

A very ugly disease bringing the world such beautiful love! I can't help but think this is true in so many ways about our group and all the love and ways it showed us to continue living.

Acknowledgments

Beautifully and happily edited by Jamie Valderrama. I am forever grateful for your expertise, time and encouragement.

Preface: Book Vision and Purpose

Rationale

The purpose of this book is to help young adults (approximately 16 to 26) cope with the unique issues they face as they navigate the world after they have been diagnosed with cancer. I've been a licensed clinical social working counseling pediatric and young adult cancer patients and their families for over 25 years. I have been an oncology social worker at University Medical Center, in Tucson Arizona, Massachusetts General Hospital in Boston, and creating and facilitating Candlelighters's of Southern Arizona Community Support Group. Throughout that time, I realized there was a dearth of information pertaining to addressing the special needs to young adults with cancer. General counseling techniques, etc. are not well suited to this group because of their developmental age, as well as their treatment team being either adult or pediatric. These young adults are already dealing with issues as to the transition from a child to an adult, dealing with issues of appearance, sexuality, struggling with dating, how they are perceived by peers/kids/adults/society/etc. This book uniquely addresses these issues because it combines multidimensional support to the young adults by creating a community. This community allows them to openly express their cancer experiences, the emotional attached to their experience and provides ongoing support in their everyday lives. It allows to address the developmental issues they are addressing in their daily lives. Creating this type of support group in communities across the United States is the foundation of meeting the needs of YA with cancer. This book highlights options and important elements in elevating existing groups and creating new ones. Each chapter has evidence and concrete tools to address the needs of YA with cancer.

My Experience

When I was obtaining my master of social work at Arizona State University, I applied for a clinical oncology traineeship through the American Cancer Society. I was fortunate to have been selected for this specialized training.

While completing my internship at the Arizona Cancer Center, I found a pressing need for a support group for young adult patients who were parents. I researched, created and facilitated a four-session group for families whose parents had cancer. I found a pattern with patients whereby many sought advice on how to parent while going through treatment. Once I recognized the common theme, I knew I needed to create a support group. After completing the entire process, including research, design, recruitment, training of medical staff for facilitating family sessions and the actual implementation, it was clear that support groups for cancer patients are invaluable in their healing.

In my past 20 years of oncology social work, specifically pediatric bone marrow transplantation and adult oncology at two well-known hospitals, Massachusetts General Hospital and University Medical Center in Tucson, Arizona I have become an experienced group facilitator. Working at Arizona State University School of Social Work for the past 15 years as a Faculty Instructor, I have found the theoretical basis on the effectiveness of group work.

As a contracted oncology social work facilitator in the community for the past 4 years, I have established an innovative and comprehensive community support group for young adults with cancer. This is an innovative approach that meets the needs of these young adults. The community support group framework fulfills the needs of young adults by meeting many of their underserved emotional needs. This includes the group itself, the social gatherings, the resources available as well as promoting post-traumatic growth. My experience in oncology, researching the needs of YA and formulating this community support group is a valuable tool for oncology professionals.

Because of the power of healing I have witnessed in facilitating this group, I was drawn to create this book to share my knowledge and to inspire young adults' voices to be heard to encourage others around the United States.

This book is an effective manual for oncology social workers and other oncology multidisciplinary members to create support groups specifically for the young adult population. This manual can be used as a teaching tool for interns and students. It can also be beneficial to clinicians that have years of experience.

As an oncology social worker, I am honored to facilitate this group. I have learned an invaluable amount of information from the voices of the young adult members of this group. I am honored that they shared their insight with me as well as their desire to help other young adults diagnosed with cancer.

Basis

In the social work profession, we highly value finding solutions for unmet needs in the community and providing necessary support. Once I realized the themes of my patients, I knew I needed to dedicate my time to creating a comprehensive support for them. In Chapter 1, I verify the research from a literature review of young adults with cancer and their unmet needs. Within the chapter, I develop the developmental themes that need to be addressed, specifically, with a support group community model. This module I have created and piloted for the past 4 years in Tucson, Arizona.

Collaborating with oncology specialists at national conferences I have been inspired to share my experience so that we can elevate comprehensive care to young adults with cancer. This book is the foundation of developing the next level of psychosocial care, particularly for young adults.

Aims of This Book

The aim is to have a comprehensive account of relevant research, issues and implementation of a young adult oncology community support group. This book is valuable to field instructors, clinicians from various backgrounds (social work, psychology, child life, psychology), students from these professions as well as professors from these disciplines. It is also useful for young adults with cancer and their loved ones.

Utilization of This Book

The book flows well from chapter to chapter. Developing educational insight throughout the book. It can also be utilized as a manual, just reading the relevant chapters to the needs of the readers. It is relevant to hospitals that provide oncology care for young adults. It can be a standard reference book for work in groups, but it also has benefits for individual work with young adults.

This book, especially Chapters 4 and 5, had insight and qualitative data from young adult members. Their voices can provide insight to their experiences. It can also be inspiring for patients fighting cancer.

I hope that this book is the foundation for more research, interventions and supportive care for young adults with cancer.

1 Developmental Issues for Young Adults With Cancer

Introduction

A diagnosis of cancer is trauma in someone's life. Cancer has negative connotations and is a scary prognosis to receive. Cancer usually involves some form of surgery with months of treatment. Most cancer patients have to put their "normal" life on hold until they're in remission. And for the majority of patients, they have to make lifelong changes in their lives because of the changes cancer causes, both physically and psychosocially. The physical growth is due to the cancer itself as well as the treatments. Some treatments stunt growth and can cause many physical changes. Throughout treatment, protocols can make some major changes in appearance. During this time of identity, it can be traumatic changes for the young adults. For example, weight gain and loss due to steroids can be devastating to self-esteem. Psychosocially leaving school, community and family to survive cancer can be very isolating. Young adults miss out on relationships and exploration of normal developmental milestones.

In the United States, approximately 80,000 young adults are diagnosed with cancer. It is evident in practice and research that this population is underserved and is in great need of psychosocial support. Young adults experience higher levels of psychosocial distress and, "yet their psychosocial needs are often not recognized or met" (Kay, Juth, Silver, & Sender, 2019, p. 502). This psychosocial distress comes out in so many ways that affect them from moving on from cancer patient to cancer survivor. Young adults must depend on their parents and caregivers during treatment which can influence dynamics within the family system. Because cancer requires such long and difficult treatment, it is considered a chronic illness. Oncology social workers must provide comprehensive care for these underserved cancer patients since their needs are so critical in this age group. This book focuses on an effective way to provide support. As an oncology social worker for the past 20 years, I have been able to experience the benefits of facilitating a support group. It is especially relevant to meet the needs of young adults as it is therapeutic in nature with the addition of peer connection and support. Many times I have observed psychosocial needs of patients and find the best way to address them is in a group setting. It is especially relevant for young adults with cancer because just being a member addresses many developmental milestones that they need to move on from cancer. "There is a need for novel support mechanisms for the very young adult's patients" (Kumar & Schapira, 2013, p. 1757). I strongly believe that the creation of a community support group meets the needs of young adults facing or surviving cancer. This book is dedicated for implementing support groups to meet this need.

Cancer and Adolescent Identity Formation

During the transitional stage from adolescence to young adulthood, the concept of self is evolving. While young adults develop their identity, the cancer can influence this progress negatively or put it on hold while fighting the disease. "AYAs with cancer face normative developmental challenges including autonomy building, identity formation and independence seeking" (Kay et al., 2019, p. 503). Going through this development requires self-awareness which is often both exciting and challenging as young adulthood is marked by physical and emotional developmental growth. "Identity formation is the most important task adolescent and emerging adults have to deal with" (Crocetti, Scrignaro, Sica, & Magrin, 2012, p. 732). Thus, the overwhelming theme of young adulthood is identity formation—a concept that crosses all aspects of the individual. As young adults progress along these years, they try new things, take new challenges and learn from mistakes. Their identity is consistently being molded through experiences on multiple facets of self, such as personality, education and relationships. It is through their likes and dislikes, independence and dependence, trial and error that evolve their individual self and determine who they will become. As young adults progress, their main influence transitions from immediate family to peers, pushing independence on a developmental rollercoaster that is both exciting and challenging. Unfortunately, the diagnosis of cancer during this stage can potentially interrupt this independent development and derail this process of self-identity as they often become totally dependent on their parents (or caregivers). "to reconstruct their identities by incorporating their experience as cancer survivors" (Kumar & Schapira, 2013, p. 1755). Young adults going through cancer often lose contact with the majority of their "healthy" friends as diagnosis and treatment pull them off the ride that their peers are all on, leading to potential trauma and developmental delays of self. It is hoped, in this book, to understand the development of the self, the impact of cancer on that development and how a support group can provide support and the opportunity to get back on that rollercoaster when dealing with cancer.

Physical Growth Considerations

The stages of adolescence and young adulthood are physiologically characterized by rapid development in the brain and body via puberty and cognitive development (This varies based on age and medical background). In this context, of young adults with cancer, it is imperative to acknowledge that the diagnosis of as well as the treatment can impair this development and have immediate and long-term side effects, such as depression, anxiety, loneliness and fear of relapse. These emotional side effects can negatively impair their quality of life. In addition to these profound emotional side effects, there can be persistent physical ones. These include sensitivity to foods, delayed physical growth, negative fertility and continued exhaustion. Some young adults have permanent hearing loss and structural changes to their physical body, from the cancer itself and the treatment. Young adults must be informed of issues that can occur physically. From an oncology social work perspective, it is evident that patients do not always process this information. These patients may be so ill after being misdiagnosed that their treatment starts pretty immediately after diagnosis. Honesty and transparency of these potential physiological and psychological issues must be addressed with the young adult patient. Oncology healthcare professionals must be diligent to bring up this information throughout diagnosis, treatment and survivorship. As the patients' brains are developing and are affected by the trauma of cancer, it must be revisited for ongoing support. Many times, this is due to the rapid progression of diagnosis to treatment, leading to the young adult patient not having time to discuss the physical complications and interruptions in normal development but rather just fighting to be alive. That being said, even if the oncology teams do address these physical and psychological issues, the young adult patient is so focused on survival that many times, they do not process this additional information.

Due to this lack of processing the negative potentiality of the treatment, many of the young adults that attend these support groups have shared that they didn't look at the long-range outcomes such as preserving their eggs or sperm for later in life—issues that are real and imminent in their daily "survivorship" from cancer.

Another key concept that is commonly discussed in support group is living with the physical changes that cancer has brought. For some, it can be evident to all (a loss of a limb), whereas for others it's a change in hair texture and color, or a scar from surgery or a port. These physical changes, brought on from cancer, are physical issues that affect their emotional well-being. It is important to recognize these changes and validate how they are feeling about these physical changes. Most significant is the connection between these physical cancer changes and how it impacts mental health. It also affects the self-awareness developing for these young adults. It's a new concept in their being that they need to process as they are discovering who they are and now with the effects of cancer.

Emotional Developmental Considerations

A recurrent theme in the young adult support group is the challenge of processing the emotional impact of the cancer diagnosis and treatment. Many put that work aside because they are unsure they would even survive, some shared that they were not sure that they wanted to survive. Reasons for this can be complex—feeling physically or emotionally so bad you don't want to live anymore, the guilt felt for negatively impacting their family or just the exhaustion from diagnosis and treatment. This realization of eminent death is profound and froze, for many, any thought of a future. Ultimately, this point of view, which many within the group could relate to, allowed them to put their feelings of change, survivorship and moving forward on hold. Then, when they became "cured," all the emotional experiences emerged as they were trying to "live their normal" life. Some young adults did understand that they needed to process these emotional realizations of the negative impact of their diagnosis and treatment but were too overwhelmed with the side effects of treatment to do this. Others expressed that they wanted to talk to someone, but felt guilty bringing it up with their loved ones, who were sad, overwhelmed and also just trying to emotionally survive. They felt like keeping the emotional impact within, away from their parents, allowing their parents to be protected. They felt guilt about taking their parents away from siblings and their lives so bringing up their emotional concerns would just be too much for their parents to handle. It was their way to have some control in an uncontrollable situation thus allowing them to protect their loved ones. A final aspect of not processing the emotional trauma of cancer was that they didn't feel like they had an outlet. When asked, the young adults felt like the oncology social workers were really just there for their parents and not for them. One way to address this is to offer a group setting where the facilitator can be the social worker for the participants. It can allow them to have a space to share these thoughts and emotions. Another idea would be to clarify the role of the social worker and confidentiality as it pertains to the medical setting and the families. A clear explanation of the role of social work and allow them to have their own, or clarify that the social worker is there for them for counseling.

In my oncology experience, I have heard from patients that despite their decision to "not address" the emotional impact of their cancer, it came up in all aspects of their life and therefore they found the support group to be a protected, safe time to process those unprocessed emotions. Perhaps, the most profound part of a support group is that many of the young adults who have therapists and mental health doctors, still regularly attend, despite their integration into the mental health system. This highlights the need for each facility and community to provide a structured support group for young adults. The connection of sharing and supporting is like no other support and one that is life changing in young adults healing from cancer. It is within these groups that they share their commonalities, recognize that they are not alone, process the trauma and emotionally heal.

As a facilitator of a young adult group, the atmosphere of a group setting is profound in their survivorship. The fact that they can connect to other young adults helps negate the feelings of isolation and depression—they are not the only ones going through the experience. This is important because in the clinical setting, they are surrounded by adults or in most cases pediatrics as they are treated, rarely meeting people their own age. This is just another aspect of why they are underserved in their care. It is within these facilitated groups, surrounded by their peers, that some of the most therapeutic interventions happen between group members.

Accessibility of these young adult support groups is vital. The following chapters will highlight not only the connections that occur in a face-to-face group but also those connections that stem from social media. "The accessibility of SM (social media) makes it an inviting option for connecting with others, particularly for individual who are geographically or socially isolated" (Shensa et al., 2020, p. 43). The incorporation of social media is particularly relevant with this population for the following reasons. Firstly, it's the most common way they communicate. Secondly, many are unable to attend a live session (due to the immune suppressed protective orders). Thirdly, many support group participants are admitted to the hospital. And lastly, it is common to have chemo treatment side effects that prevent them from driving (examples are migraines, nausea and colds). These issues can prevent regular group attendance but allowing for SM connection can negate these obstacles and is an important aspect of a successful young adult support group. The group is a foundation for them to connect as a community. To have that continuous support needed to get them through the process of cancer and becoming an adult. The support group is the foundation of connections within the community that you create.

Another important aspect that needs to be addressed is the geographical location of the group. What other support systems are available for young adults? Does the group design address the needs in the community? If you live in a large rural area, sometimes financial support is not possible for participants. They might not have enough money for gas or reliable transportation, and or weather conditions may prevent them from attending. By incorporating the SM option, it allows for this population to always be connected to their young adult community support group. It is a key component to consider as you develop your group. It also is the foundation for participants to connect outside of the group. Knowing they can reach out and meet up with their new community is a relief. In our group, members have become friends, volunteered together and reached out during a difficult time. It becomes another community support and provides them a source of social connections which is a foundation for their developmental stage.

Emotional Themes

The emotional development that occurs throughout young adulthood is dynamic. Going through cancer, only makes that development more complicated. The group setting allows these young adults with cancer to have a platform to share their emotional progression. This self-awareness is important to acknowledge so that they can articulately express their feelings and the group facilitator can identify new dynamics that emerge. It's an ongoing lesson in their emotional needs and development with the group setting providing a venue to shift the perspective of negative emotional themes to positive. "Transition periods can also function as turning points, providing opportunities for change from negative to more positive developmental pathways in subsequent developmental periods" (Scales et al., 2015, p. 153). When sharing their emotional processing of the effects of cancer with their peers, they allow the feedback and connection to "normalize" their experience in relation to the cancer. Sometimes it happens immediately and sometimes it takes a while to process depending on the group dynamics. But it is through this disclosure that the facilitator can glean emotional themes and effectively guide the group forward.

Emotions About Treatment

The emotional trauma of survivors has no defined timeline and can be just as raw for an individual 5 years out as for one 5 months out. Sharing their stories with one another is a profound process that peels away layers of emotional residue. An example of how this happens is when a new member comes, regardless of time within the group, there is always a fresh introduction from all. Repeatedly hearing the same introductions triggers emotions that may still be present. Many veteran members say that there is a new element or perspective they gain when listening, and it is through the safety of the group setting that they are able to disclose more and more.

Some of the young adults who attend support groups have shared that they were not able to comprehend the effects during treatment. Many of the continued issues that come up in group are processing the emotional side of cancer. For example, some patients talk about how when they were diagnosed and being treated, they never wanted to bring up their intense sadness and fears so that they could protect their parents/caregivers. Some felt intense feelings of depression and or anxiety but were so focused on just surviving that they didn't have enough energy to address these emotional side effects of cancer. In addition, there are some physical changes that happen which they need to emotionally process after they have come into remission. A common issue that happens to young adults is an issue of fertility. Some young adults didn't have the option to preserve their eggs or sperm prior to treatment. Most cancer treatments cause infertility. When they were facing life or death, fertility seemed so intangible. But once they are in remission the issues come up. Unfortunately, due to time and financial concerns not all young adults are able to take precautions to preserve their eggs or sperm. This is due to lack of time, and financial restrictions. But years after in group, these issues are real and imminent in their daily "survivorship" from cancer. It might be effective to provide some additional referrals, and or psychoeducational sessions with experts in the field, so the young adults have more choices and education about this pressing issue. It would be a way for them to be able to ask general questions and know where to go for support. Referrals are always the basis of a social work tool, but the group setting is also an ideal setting for quests speakers.

The complexity of their emotions are multifaceted and cover past, present and future as they process where they were, where they are and where they will go both personally and with their loved ones.

Another powerful dynamic that occurs within a positively functioning group is their desire to give back. They want to support others by providing a positive framework for how to go through this and find meaning. Over the past years, some sessions have impressed me; the young adults have put aside their pressing issues when a new member comes in. They are able to give back and advice even when they are seeking it. They want their experience to mean something, to teach others who have not experienced this and to help those who will—thus the creation of this book.

Post-Traumatic Growth

Becoming a member of a group is an example of post-traumatic growth. Through their ability to positively process their trauma, many young adult survivors are motivated to take their experience and give back. "Post-traumatic growth occurs when the awareness of vulnerability is accompanied y an augmented sense of becoming more capable and self-reliant and when individuals are able to find new meanings in life and social relationships" (Arpawong, Oland, Milam, Ruccione, & Meeske, 2013, p. 1002). They are asked by those medical professionals who shared their journey to encourage and provide hope for other young adults going through cancer. Some even go beyond and continue to inspire through community organizations and volunteering at camps or events that they attended while they were in treatment.

Other young adults' team up with fundraising. They raise money by running a race, or sharing their story to elicit donations. A few even choose career paths that allow them to give back to others facing cancer such as social service or medical, inspired to live a life that is meaningful and dedicated to service. On a personal level, many find new meaning in their life, an appreciation of gratitude and perspective that they never had before.

Survivorship

The relief and excitement of finally being cancer free opens a new phase of lifelong survivorship. Thinking about the "normal" developmental milestones that young adults progress through, it is evident that many of these milestones were not explored due to cancer diagnosis and treatment. Therefore, the support group provides an environment to process the loss of these milestones in a safe, connecting way. Addressing the grief over the loss of old self, missed opportunities and certainty of health highlight the trauma that carries over. It's a safe place to express their sadness over these losses. Developing new friendships, determining when and if they should disclose their cancer history as well as the impact that cancer has made on who they have become are very real. Acknowledging this is important to the healing of these young adult survivors as well as the realization that survivorship becomes a foundation from which they build the rest of their lives. Being able to share these feelings in a place where they feel safe and understood is very important.

Cancer Support Groups

Oncology support groups regularly address these compound issues for young adults with cancer. Understanding the developmental stage allows for this comprehension. To alleviate the impact from cancer treatment, the development of a young adult support group is key, "social support has a profound and far-reaching impact on mental and physical health and health behavior," Shensa et al., 2020, p. 38). Acknowledging that cancer treatment on young adults is profound, validates their experience and allows them to connect and find support from others that really know what it's like. The healing benefit of a support group for young adults is the interaction and connections they make between themselves. As a facilitator to be able to witness, the support and profound connection are the most beneficial part. The way in which they give and receive support is therapeutic. In all my years of education, I have never learned more about the intimate struggle of cancer but by this group. In terms of educating an oncology social worker, this facilitation can be enlightening to the experience of cancer, something magical and profound that occurs in each group. Not only about surviving cancer but also about the meaning of life and all the human dynamics of relationships.

Integration of Developmental Issues Consistently Within the Group Community

As stated in research by (Zebrack et al., 2016, p. 1941) . . . they (social workers) are doing less with respect to conducting follow-up and re-evaluations of psychosocial treatment plans. This follow-up is key to the success of a group. By consistently evaluating the feedback of the group, it provides a roadmap on what issues need to be addressed, as well as validates the groups thoughts as to where they are at. It is important to integrate breaks where the young adults can just have fun and not talk about "deep" issues. Some sessions can be utilized for bonding and relaxing, especially after some emotional challenging ones. It is a key component of having a group. Sometimes it is member initiated; we do questions in a box and sometimes those questions are you afraid of dying. Sometimes the questions are what is your favorite desert? That is a part of group processing and the magical process that goes on in a group. Acknowledging and allowing for breaks are a key lesson in their lives. The young adults also like trying new things like yoga and/or meditation. Learning new skills is a key element of the group that allows for growth and variety. Zebrak's work encourages social workers to research their work so they can collaborate in professional realms with current research to provide the best care for cancer patients and provide evidence-based practice. "These findings have the practical implications, suggesting the importance of interventions aimed at promoting critical evaluations of identity alternatives in order to support adolescents and emerging adults in finding a set of fulfilling commitments" (Crocetti et al., 2012, p. 745). In order to help these young adults affected by cancer, the foundation of developmental milestones, particularly identity formation, must be the basis of the work. Keeping these developmental milestones at the forefront of the group structure helps to keep the intervention focused and relevant. "Oncology social work has emerged as a specialized discipline in which social workers provide a ranch of psychosocial services to individuals, groups and communities interacting with cancer care" (Pockett, Dzidowska, & Hobbs, 2015, p. 583). What makes this group so healing is a foundation in social work where many dynamics of life are integrated. Therefore, providing a basis for a community is a key element in creating your group. Starting where the members are, allowing them to create and impact the flow of the group, leads to greater connection.

In the following chapters, ideas and specific interventions will be described so that the development of each group is based in effective treatment. The advantage of social work is that there are many creative facets to address the same underlying issues. Starting at basic developmental stages is fundamental in providing a safe and encouraging space for young adult cancer survivors. Based on the research, the themes identified in the following group structures will address the needs and development of young adults. "The changes are so significant that emerging adults need substantial supports to navigate the transition successfully. Emerging adults with disabilities or chronic health conditions require more support to maximize their potential development during EA (Emerging Adults)" (Wood et al., 2018). Because of the variety in social work, the different ways to impact people formatting the group under this basis is key. Allowing to try art work and different means of therapeutic intervention keep the members engaged and excited to participate. A secondary benefit of the group is that of the clinical social worker. They learn different techniques and issues that can help other group members or their individual counseling with cancer patients. An oncology social worker that facilitates groups is a stronger, well-experienced social worker and helps the individual and group work they provide. I always thank the young adults and remind them how much they are helping me in the work that I do by sharing their experience.

References

Arpawong, T. E., Oland, A., Milam, J. E., Ruccione, K., & Meeske, K. A. (2013). Post-traumatic growth among an ethnically diverse sample of adolescent and young adult cancer survivors. *Psycho-Oncology, 22*, 2235–2244. https://doi.org/10.1002/pon.3286

Crocetti, E., Scrignaro, M., Sica, L., & Magrin, S. (2012). Correlates of identity configurations: Three studies with adolescent and emerging adult cohorts. *Journal of Youth and Adolescence, 41*(6), 732–748.

Kay, J. S., Juth, V., Silver, R., & Sender, L. (2019). Support and conflict in relationships and psychological health in adolescents and young adults with cancer. *Journal of Health Psychology, 24*(4), 502–517.

Kumar, A. R., & Schapira, L. (2013). The impact of intrapersonal, interpersonal, and community factors on the identity formation of young adults with cancer: A qualitative study: Identity formation of young adults with cancer. *Psycho-oncology* (Chichester, England), *22*(8), 1753–1758.

Lazard, A. J., Saffer, A., Horrell, L., Benedict, C., & Love, B. (2019). Peer-to-peer connections: Perceptions of a social support app designed for young adults with cancer. *Psycho-oncology* (Chichester, England), *29*(1), 173–181.

Pockett, R., Dzidowska, M., & Hobbs, K. (2015). Social work intervention research with adult cancer patients: A literature review and reflection on knowledge-building for practice. *Social Work in Health Care*, *54*(7), 582–614.

Scales, P. C., Benson, P. L., Oesterle, S., Hill, K. G., Hawkins, J. D., & Pashak, T. J. (2015). The dimensions of successful young adult development: A conceptual and measurement framework. *Applied Developmental Science*, *20*(3), 150–174. https://doi.org/10.1080/10888691.2015.1082429

Shensa, A., Sidani, J. E., Escobar-Viera, C. G., Switzer, G. E., Primack, B. A., & Choukas-Bradley, S. (2020). Emotional support from social media and face-to-face relationships: Associations with depression risk among young adults. *Journal of Affective Disorders*, *260*, 38–44.

Wood, D., Crapnell, T., Lau, L., Bennett, A., Lotstein, D., Ferris, M., & Kuo, A. (2018). Emerging adulthood as a critical stage in the life course. In N. Halfon, C. Forrest, R. Lerner, & E. Faustman (Eds.), *Handbook of life course health development*. Cham: Springer.

Zebrack, B., Kayser, K., Padgett, L., Sundstrom, L., Jobin C., Nelson, K., & Fineberg, I. C. (2016). Institutional capacity to provide psychosocial oncology support services: A report from the Association of Oncology Social Work. *Cancer*, *122*, 1937–1945.

2 Supporting Young Adults in a Closed Group Format
Insights From Practice at Massachusetts General Hospital

Introduction

Massachusetts General Hospital (MGH) is the epitome of social work integration in medical care. Every department has a staff of social workers who specialize in their field. The basis of comprehensive care is that the social work presence is valued, respected and appreciated at every level. Since 1944, MGH's social work department has evolved, and it is now the ideal collaborative structure of medical treatment and social work interventions. The MGH cancer center is designed around the most comprehensive care of oncology specialists and social workers that provide individual interventions for patients, group designs and integrative support for patients and families.

I had the honor to work at MGH on the colorectal adult oncology team, I was able to attend Swartz Rounds. I had the amazing opportunity to listen and reflect on important issues in patient care. The mission of Swartz Rounds is to allow open discussion on the emotional and social issues around care of cancer patients. The panel is a multidisciplinary team openly discussing current care issues around how to provide comprehensive care to patients. The invaluable openness of panel and participants is enlightening for professionals. To be able to take the time to discuss these significant issues that teams don't always have time to process allows a deeper understanding into our own professional development. We discussed what it was like to feel connected to a patient our own age and how it impacted our care. We talked about how it emotionally felt to have a patient die. It was the first time in my profession I was able to discuss these emotional issues with my colleagues. After attending a few rounds, I was asked to participate as a facilitator discussing young adult patients. Some of my present colleagues were on the panel and in the audience and the emotional connections that occurred have shaped who I am today.

In 2003, those young adult Swartz Rounds inspired me to create and facilitate a young adult cancer support group. Because I was one of the newest social workers at MGH and on the oncology team, I decided to review the structure of a group that was completed a few years earlier. I was motivated to incorporate the issues presented at Swartz Rounds around the young adult cancer patients we provided care for. Therefore, I used the structure of the group another MGH social worker had used but with the determination to focus the group on the issues of Swartz Rounds that became relevant in my work with young adults. I felt that a group would be the best setting to learn from the young adults and allow them a much-needed opportunity to process with others of the same age. "Overall, 39.6% of AYA patients responding to the survey 6–14 months after diagnosis reported needing some type of health services with the most common service needed being mental health (35.2%) followed by support group 17.7%)" (Prasad et al., 2014, p. 734). The purpose of this book is to meet the needs of this underserved population. The foundation of these ideas will be the basis of protocols on the most effective way to meet these identified needs of young adults with cancer.

Group Structure

The oncology social workers all indicated they had patients within the age range of young adults, 18–25. Each was able to educate and refer their patients to participate in the group. To be included in the group, they needed to contact me and complete an initial assessment. I knew that it would be beneficial for them to be able to ask specific questions, which would guide me in understanding what was and was not significant to them. I also realized that it was important to center the group around age and not their diagnosis. Consequently, this became one of the biggest challenges when facilitating the group. In collaborating with the brain tumor social worker, who made a referral, I was not prepared with the right skills on how to facilitate a group with someone with a brain tumor. When it was his turn to speak, it was very long and unfocused. As soon as it was identified, I met with the social worker to get some skills on how to address so that everyone in the group had the same amount of time to share. At that point, the brain tumor patients had an online facilitated support group run by the social worker, which was a good setting. At the same time, allowing him to participate provided a valuable example. Another issue is that some discussions took longer, due to different treatment protocols. When all group members have the same cancer, many things are familiar to the group and take less time about the education and more about the personal experience. It is a dynamic to consider when planning a group and how to provide ample time and education within the group. It should be noted that the community was taken into account when creating this group. MGH has a very comprehensive social work presence in the cancer center. They have social workers present in the library to assist patients, caregivers and extended families in collecting resources. They have ongoing weekly drop-in groups. Some of these groups included mindful meditation, visualization, specific groups for particular diagnosis and educational and psychoeducational ongoing groups. In addition, these groups collaborate with other professionals, nutritionists and psychologists. MGH also offers integrative health options, such as exercise and relaxation. Each specialty has a team of social workers which are a valuable part of the multidisciplinary team. Taking this setting into account was a huge guide for the structure of the group. For these reasons, I created a closed six-week group in which participants had to meet for approval and agree to attend all of the sessions.

Initial Intake

The initial intake was a short one-page interview. Some were completed over the phone while others were completed at the cancer center. It was a way for the facilitator to get to know the participants and their needs. It allowed them to be in a comfortable setting and be able to ask any questions they had about group. It was also a way to individually go over the expectations of the group and the structure. It felt like the perfect way to explain what would happen in group. It also allowed for relationship building between participants and the facilitator, since many of the participants were coming from other parts of the cancer center.

One-page open-ended intake

1) Referring Social Worker – this was significant because it was stated at the initial intake that collaboration between the facilitator and social worker would only occur if there were any concerning issues that the referring social worker would need to follow up with (social issues, financial or presenting psychological issues).
2) Introduction

   a. Type of Cancer
   b. Type of Treatment
   c. Ever attended a group before? What was that experience like?
   d. Where are you in treatment and/or follow-up
   e. Type of support already utilized within MGH.
   f. What do you want to share with me?
   g. What are you looking to get out of group?

Each interview lasted from thirty minutes to an hour. The group started about 2 weeks after the last interview. At that point, the group was closed to participants. Every patient that had an interview was an appropriate match for participation in the group. The total participation for the first session was eight young adults. It should be noted that some patients referred were not interested in the group or did not contact the group facilitator. It is also significant to mention if the young adults referred were at the later part of the age cutoff, they were parents and did not feel it was an appropriate agenda for their needs as parents facing cancer. If all the young adults had been parents, we would have shifted the group to a parenting while going through cancer.

Group Agenda

For the 6-week group, each session was detailed and revolved around milestones of young adults facing cancer. The group took place at the MGH Library conference room in the early evening from 6 to 7:30 pm. This room was chosen in part so that the table was big enough to incorporate room for completing art projects around the night's varied themes. The reason multiple themes were incorporated was because "young adults enacted their beliefs and behaviors within the process of supportive care" (Soanes et al., 2015).

Week 1-Introduction
Week 2-Treatment
Week 3-Self Image
Week 4-Relationships
Week 5-Cancer Concerns and the Future
Week 6-Summary and Closure

Each session I was the facilitator and I also had a social work intern who attended to observe the process of group. MGH always encouraged the teaching environment for young adults. There were sessions during the day between the MSW student and I to go over how and when she would participate or lead each session. After all participants left for the evening, there would be a debriefing of the group. Group participants were not asked to complete evaluations of the group during the 6 weeks.

Week 1-Introduction

The goal of the first session was relationship building and group expectations. As the participants arrived, we had snacks on the table and had informal discussions. This is a foundation of a developmental stage, connecting with people. Once everyone was present, we had a round circle of chairs where we went through the group structure and expectations. We had a large sheet of paper that we explained was an open invite to write down things that were important to the group setting in order to establish set guidelines. Most participants had never participated in a closed support group so we were sure to emphasize confidentiality and mandated reporting as well as encourage participants to share their concerns as well as suggestions.

After the development of our group guidelines, we moved into introductions. I introduced my role as the facilitator and spoke about my prior experience in pediatric bone marrow transplantation at University Medical center in Tucson, Arizona. The MSW intern then did her introduction. From there, we asked for volunteers to introduce themselves, handing out an idea sheet to help with their introduction that included name, age, diagnosis, who they lived with, what they did currently for school or employment, interests and something special about them. They were encouraged to answer only what they felt comfortable with and were free to introduce themselves in anyway. In terms of the agenda, this took a lot more time than expected but it gave them a solid foundation of sharing to build upon comfortable conversation as we moved forward. We concluded the meeting with an overview of the themes that we would address in the following weeks.

Week 2-Treatment

All the young adults returned for the second session. They were more comfortable and were able to have small discussions between themselves before the start of group. It validated that the relationship building of the first group had been successful. I reminded the group of the expectations that they had created in the prior meeting and moved into the week's theme, having them discuss the treatment that they had been through. What we discovered was not necessarily talk of treatment but rather discussion about the pre-diagnosis symptoms, trials and tribulations. There was great detail shared about the way in which they were diagnosed and how emotional that was. Once everyone shared, they then moved into treatment, asking each other questions or sharing similar experiences.

In debriefing, we realized that the discussion was a lot more emotional than expected and that the "treatment" session ended up being more about the experience prior to diagnosis and leading up to treatment which was enlightening. This information was not only vital to processing for the group but educated us, the clinicians, on what impacted these young adults.

Clinical Decision-Flexibility

When I was doing my weekly hour in the oncology library, a young adult happened to come in and ask about the group. He really wanted to come but was completing treatment and would only be able to attend the third week. I definitely struggled with this as the initial setup was that participants needed to commit to all of the sessions. At the same time, this was a young adult who really wanted to participate. I collaborated with the other social workers and finally came to the decision that he could attend. The session was actually amazing. This male young adult had an amazingly positive affect on the group. They really bonded with him despite the fact that he was only going to attend one session and were inspired by him. The lesson learned was that being flexible was beneficial to the participants as well as the leaders. And the fact that he wanted to participant it must have met a need in his healing.

Week 3-Self Image

Week 3's session was the one that we had the additional participant attend so we took a brief time to allow him to introduce himself. Despite our concern, it was amazing how easily these now connected young adults accepted him. Because this week was about self-image, which is a major issue during this developmental age, we had the young adults share the physical changes that happened to them due to cancer. We used art for this session to help them process. They chatted while doing the art which was beneficial for bonding as well as interpersonal skills. We had them draw themselves both before and then after cancer diagnosis. While they worked, they asked each other questions and gave each other support. We observed that they liked being able to create with art and that it was a helpful way to facilitate relationship building. It was also a fun and safe place for them to focus on creativity and commonality. Once they were done, we then had them share their two self-images, comparing the changes pre- and post-cancer. There was a lot of support for one another and relief in hearing others experiencing the same feelings. There was a lot about the emotional attitude that was caused by the physical changes. A strong underlying theme was loss.

In the debriefing after, we determined the activity was therapeutic, fun and a powerful way to express their feelings through art. It also introduced an additional tool for them as a coping skill. It highlighted the effectiveness of art therapy, adding to my own toolbox of resources that I would share in the future with young adults.

Week 4-Relationships

Week 4 focused on relationships. We gave the young adults paper and had them illustrate, anyway that they wanted, significant relationships they had through their cancer. They could use words, colors or designs representing friends, family, medical professionals, therapists and significant others.

Once they completed their representation of these relationships, we then had a group discussion sharing how these relationships changed as they moved through their treatment. Week 4 highlighted a group that had bonded, were supporting one another and needed less guidance from the facilitators. They disclosed with one another that in order to protect many of their relationships, they had often not been fully forthcoming or authentic in what they were feeling and going through. This group setting provided them the safe place to share this commonality and reinforce that they were not alone in their feelings and behaviors.

Week 5-Cancer Concerns and the Future

Week 5 delved into how cancer had affected their personalities, their plans and how they would move forward. What was expected to be discussed and what actually was revealed was quite different. There was a lot of disclosure about their concerns for future reproduction. "Our results indicate that cancer survivors with an unfulfilled desire to have children might be a particularly vulnerable group" (Ernst et al., 2020, p. 485). The fear of relapse, and grief over losing their precancer self and future. This section could have been shifted into many sessions since so many issues became present. The young adults were able to connect by having related medications and reactions, even if not exactly the same, they could relate. Fertility was not something that was specifically planned to be discussed but it was discussed first when asked about the future. The young adults talked about their precancer plans for families and then what happened to them at diagnosis. Some had been able to save eggs or sperm and somewhere not. Fertility had many emotions attached. Some were fearful of getting follow-up with an OBGYN to see if their eggs were still viable. The fear and sadness attached to this process were strong and everyone could relate even if their fertility and cancer issues were different. In reflecting the shorter discussion, it would have been helpful to have this be an open topic and maybe even some psychoeducation about fertility after cancer.

It was also evident that every young adult had anxiety and concern about their follow-up post-remission. It is a time where they challenge every cough, pain or feeling tired, afraid that the cancer is back. This is an everyday issue that eases with time, but it is present and the awareness that cancer can come back can be limiting in the future. They shed some tears and connected over their follow-up days. It was also discussed grief over the changes cancer has made to their future, out of their control. Things like being a part of the military, or a pro athlete, or even a lifelong career change. This was heard in each of the young adults' experience and is relevant in moving forward. Allowing the grief of loss be present while they move forward in the future.

Week 6-Summary and Closure

Week 6 was all about celebration and closure. We ate a meal together that was donated by a local restaurant. The members had time to chat in groups and reflect about what they had experienced overall in the group. We gave everyone the opportunity to share what it was like for them to participate as well as asked about specific challenges that had surfaced for them, how they were coping with those challenges and plans for resolution. The feedback was positive despite the emotional elements that occurred and members developed strong enough connections with one another that they exchanged contact information. We encouraged them to keep in touch, as the group was just the foundation of support moving forward.

Reflecting on this last group meeting, I regret not utilizing a written group assessment. I feel like the young adults may have been able to share more about their experience if they had a chance to write vs the verbal format of the last group. I could have asked for concrete feedback on their transformation and given them a chance to more deeply evaluate their experience which we were not able to do because of time. Because of this, I may have missed critical feedback to take forward from this group. I feel that a written evaluation would have also given them an element of empowerment in contributing to the field of social work and future young adults with cancer.

Limitations of the Group

It should be stated that this structure was only used one time with nine young adults. That limits the effectiveness of this group setup. The setting was in Boston, Massachusetts and in a hospital that had a multitude of supports for cancer patients. Not only is the hospital providing comprehensive psychosocial support, within the city of Boston and the surrounding top-rated cancer centers there are a vast amount of resources. It should be noted that even within this amount of emotional support, young adults were still needing peer support groups for this underserved population. Also, there was no track or acknowledgment of cultural diversity. Another limitation was that there were no evaluations except for the discussions at the end of each group session. The last session only had a discussion of the impact of the group but there was no written documentation of the impact of the group.

Clinical Considerations

The power of this group was the commonality of cancer and their age. There were similar experiences with treatment, feelings and fears throughout each session, successfully showing that a closed short commitment support group is an effective way to provide a positive intervention for young adults with cancer. For a setting like MGH where there are a lot of additional multidisciplinary supports as well as an abundance of social work individual counseling, a closed group is a great option. It seemed like an appropriate commitment for young adults. By adding the initial intake, it provided more of a connection to the facilitator and the group atmosphere while ensuring commitment. It would also be beneficial to have a written survey that they could share experiences not willing to share through verbal communication. The survey could serve as a foundation of research. It could also be used to get them used to filling out a survey at each session so their voices are heard for evaluation. Explaining that their input is important in structuring the group as well as education professionals on the needs of young adults with cancer. This gives them a sense of purpose and a way to give back from their experience.

A key component to add would be to incorporate an evaluation. Implementing a written format that is effective would provide the facilitator a foundation for improvement from session to session as well as empower the young adults with a purpose of helping both themselves and others. In addition, this pilot highlighted the need for more in-depth coverage of topics; thus, it would be recommended to have more time and less themes.

Some considerations that might develop from this pilot:

- Ongoing short-term young adult groups that focus on condensed themes. It gives the young adults the option to go to sessions that are most relevant to them.
- Provide a short evaluation to be able to improve on sessions. It also gives the young adults pride in helping others (both other cancer survivors and clinicians).
- Have each session be longer than an hour and a half. Lots of discussion occurs, especially when there is an activity prior to the discussion.
- When social workers refer their patients, ask what they feel the most relevant needs/themes should be addressed in order to provide the most effective sessions.
- Incorporate group feedback to the sessions.
- Consider follow-up half-day sessions on popular topics. For example, conference for young adults on fertility, relationships or self-image. Providing a follow-up to a closed group ensures the continued community once the sessions are complete.
- Since the initial group years ago, young adult's dependence on social media has vastly increased. Incorporating a closed social media to provide updates and encourage the community feel within the young adult's participants.

- Bring in new social work clinicians—this is the most productive way to gain experience as a group facilitator. It allows for a manageable transition and experience for new clinicians.
- A closed group is very appealing to young adults since they have so much going on. The interventions will reach more young adults since it's less of a commitment.
- Facilitating a group is a really beneficial for interns to learn about the themes and issues for young adults with cancer. A great learning setting for interns from all disciplines.
- Think of the group as community building for them, creating a connecting support in their lives within group as well as outside of group.

References

Ernst, M., Brähler, E., Wild, P. S., Faber, J., Merzenich, H., & Beutel, M. E. (2020). The desire for children among adult survivors of childhood cancer: Psychometric evaluation of a cancer-specific questionnaire and relations with sociodemographic and psychological characteristics. *Psycho-Oncology, 29*(3), 485–492.

Prasad, P. K., Landry, I., Keegan, T. H. M., Harlan, L., Parsons, H., Lynch, C. F., . . . Wu, X.-C. (2014). Healthcare services needs and co-morbidity assessment among adolescents and young adults with cancer: The AYA Hope Study. *Blood, 124*(21), 734–734.

Soanes, L. (2015). Meeting the supportive care needs of young adults with cancer. *British Journal of Nursing, 24*(suppl. 16), S30.

3 Supporting Young Adults in a Group Format

Insights From Practice With the Candlelighters's Community

Introduction

In fall of 2015, I was offered the opportunity to create and run a support group in Tucson, Arizona for young adults with cancer. The local Candelighter's of Southern Arizona, a nonprofit that provides support to cancer patients and their families, had just received a grant to facilitate a group. Tucson is a region of the United States where there is no current support groups for teenagers and young adults with cancer (YAG). This YAG population are either seen on the adult or pediatric unit, which is a source of isolation. Many cancer patients find support when they connect with others their age either in support group or in wait and treatment rooms. Therefore, the importance of this support in Tucson was vital to the needs of the young adults. Along with Candelighter's, another local foundation, Courtney's Courage, was interested in providing a meal before each group to help provide more opportunity for relationship building. Courtney's Courage's mission is dedicated to raising funds for pediatric cancer research, specifically neuroblastoma, and to support those families whose children are suffering from cancer. With the collaboration of Candelighter's and Courtney's Courage, local social workers and myself, we have been able to meet the community needs for teenagers and young adults throughout the past 4 years. The development and support of all collaborated parts have continued to provide these young adults with a support group within a successful community that meets the needs of cancer patients throughout Tucson.

Structure Consideration

There were a lot of considerations in the process of planning the group. The primary location of young adults' treatment is at Banner University Medical Center in Tucson, so the group was to be in the hospital. The inpatient unit was the location since it would allow for young adults admitted to the hospital to have the option to participate in the group. Because of the social economic and the isolation issue for young adults, we knew we were going to provide a meal prior to the group. The significance of the dinner was to encourage young adults to come and connect with others in an informal social connection as well as ensure they had a meal. Another benefit to the meal was that the young adults got to know the founder of Courtney's Courage and learn about a foundation that was created for the founder's daughter and her fight against neuroblastoma. Over the years of this particular relationship has been influential. Some of the YAG members have been speakers are their annual golf fundraiser. They have also been interviewed and recorded for their funding video. The post-traumatic growth that the foundation's essence can be inspirational to the young adults. The support of Courney's Courage throughout the past 4 years has been an incredible benefit to the individual members and the group as a whole. The nonprofit's influence in the young adult group will be mentioned throughout this chapter.

Group was going to be once a month and in the evening, a time that newly diagnosed young adults could attend as well as active patients and survivors. The first group was conducted in the cafeteria private room, and the proceeding groups were designed from the initial meeting. One of the members suggested having it on the inpatient unit, as they had wished the group was available when they were hospitalized.

First Group

Despite the fact that I was an experienced oncology social worker, I was nervous for the first group. I had created and designed many oncology groups in my career but this one felt more crucial to succeed. The fact that both funders were parents of children who had died of cancer made it more emotional for me. Since my previous groups, I had elevated my social work practice by becoming a faculty instructor at Arizona State University. I learned the vital connection of evidence-based practice as I became involved in social work research. Therefore, every decision within the group was even more critical to provide the best support. I also knew the research showed that young adults with cancer, especially in Tucson, Arizona lacked support. I was concerned about being an outside contractor and not the oncology social worker in the treatment setting. I had a lot to prove and provide for this group to be a success. As a professional oncology social worker, I had worked through all these elements and was able to focus on the present group.

First Group Lessons

My most memorable event from the group was that one young adult was very upset as his mom made him come to group. He really didn't want to be there but by the end of group, he said, "I am so happy I came and I liked group . . . but don't tell my mom."

I utilized one of the art projects from the Mass General Group format. The hand and color in or design with color and or words about who you are. I used this as an ice breaker and a way to introduce ourselves. Some, especially the males, did not love this activity. But I guess even when an activity is not a success, it serves a purpose. We connected over the laughs of it. Also, they were able to verbalize what they liked and did not like in the group. So, throughout the past 4 years, if I design a project or activity that they don't like, we talk about the activity. The young adults are very expressive and share their input in evaluating our activities. We figure out a way to improve or change up the activity so it meets their needs. As a group facilitator, being flexible and open to change is a key component to success. It builds trust within the group.

Reflection of Lessons and Further Research Considerations

Some members that attended the first group still regularly attend 4 years later so establishing my role as a caring, understanding facilitator of the cancer process is key in the establishment of a successful group. Throughout the years of participation, I am always awed by how a member can come and even if they are the only one, they stay, share and process intense issues with me. It is through the trust and consistency established that I have had this happen, even with new members.

Another lesson I have learned is that it is important to design each group like it's the first and or last group in order to make an impact. As the facilitator, you want to influence them even if they do not return to the group community. Taking that perspective as you design each session really helps because it's foundational in social work to make every interaction meaningful and therapeutic.

I share the above thoughts because, despite being an oncology social worker and Arizona State University faculty, some of these key clinical components are not learned in books and evidence-based practice. To truly have a successful group, it's important that the facilitator can create relationships that connect with these young adults beyond the data. A group facilitator should really have specific training in oncology social work. And it is important to have an openness to adapt to where these young adults are. Some have said it really helps that I was not their team social worker because they felt they were there for their parents and not for them. It's a very interesting dynamic to discuss and look into in terms of oncology social work interventions. Is this a part of why young adults are underserved psychosocially? They feel the social worker is for their parents and not for them during treatment? Does it depend on the social worker? How do we evaluate this? It is an interesting concept to explore and to do research on since I have such great feedback from the young adults that have attended the group.

Another aspect that is very significant in a group is timing. Some participants have started group right after diagnosis. Others have come years out of survivorship. What is the influential factor in trying a support group? From what I have learned from facilitating the group is that timing is individual. This is another reason for ongoing sessions or continuous closed groups. Another component of participation is perception of their support or lack thereof. The process of referral is another consideration. Who is making the referral and how is the group explained?

Overview of Group Process and Design

As stated above, the group for the first 6 months was scheduled for once a month. Because of continued evaluation from the young adults, their participation and ideas were always considered. Not only did this shape the progression of the group, it also gave the young adults a voice so that it was tailored to their preferences. One key aspect they did not like was the schedule. Since cancer treatment and survivorship can have a multitude of negative side effects, a lot of times the young adults would plan to attend group. But for some medical reason, they were unable to come. If this happened, they would have to wait an entire month to come. So, they asked for the schedule to be changed to twice a month. This was a beneficial consideration and the attendance dramatically increased.

Three years into the group, we had one young adult relapse who had been a regular attendee. We also had two new young adults that had just been diagnosed come in. Needs for the participants' change based off of where they are but the need for support is consistent which was when I integrated Zoom for participants that wanted to attend but couldn't. We used Zoom for over a year, and it was a beneficial solution when participants were in isolation due to treatment. It connected them and allowed the young adults in group to support their members. The most effective way this worked was to pick a specific time for them to connect during the group. Often the young adult on the zoom just needed to give and update, get some support and check in. This process usually took about 20 minutes but the zoom participant had the option of participating during the entire session. This additional option of joining with Zoom allowed for more socialization and connection and is highly recommended to offer this additional technology to make the group connections stronger.

The implementation of Zoom was serendipitous when in March of 2020, COVID-19 emerged. Because we were already using this technology, it was an easy adjustment, same dates and times as planned. We were also still able to complete the pre- and post-evaluations on the chat section of the zoom template. I was able to cut and paste the responses into my group research. Zoom also proved beneficial in the chat section where the young adults were able to communicate their personal answers to one another in private. Ironically, Zoom was instrumental for these young adults due to the global epidemic and the additional support it spurred with the group members. In addition, between the regularly scheduled support Zoom groups, I added short psychoeducational Zooms. Some of these were visualization, body scan and stretch classes. These additional Zooms were 30 minutes in time and without pre- and post-evaluations. I implemented these because the young adults were talking about the epidemic taking always their self-care and supports, such as exercising at the gym, going out and socializing. So, they asked to learn more concrete coping skills. This was not something that had been requested in the past and it was comforting to know that they felt confident enough to ask and identify their current needs in this uncertain time.

Communication

When the group was created, all correspondence was through email. The referrals were also coming through email. The hospital social workers in town would give the young adults my name and number or email me their information.

We then moved to texting instead of email, since young adults were not dependable emailers. At that point, I created a closed Facebook page, since I was also giving them information about local and national cancer supports as well as financial aid and scholarships. Over the years, I have started collaborating with other institutions, specifically Dana Farber Cancer Institute in Boston, who has an extensive young adult program. I share a lot of their podcasts and events. I also belong to some cancer groups, Cancer Sucks, and Massachusetts General Hospital Cancer events. Topics range from social work issues, to financial education, sexuality and of course, cancer. I figure the more reliable information the group can have access to the better. Most of them read and find the information helpful. I also provide local Tucson events on this page. Some young adults that have not attended for a while still like to be on the Facebook page for all of the resources.

As of present, I have a group text reminding them of group times and schedules. If they can't make it, I encourage them to send an update on how they are doing.

Individual Support

If one participant is having a particularly hard time, I ask if they want more support. Sometimes they just want me to text them during the week to see how they are doing. Sometimes it maybe a phone call. Some of the young adults connect with me so that they can process personal issues because they are not willing to go to an outside counselor. In that case, I have met alone with young adults for additional support. Just reminding them that I am there is important. Some have taken up the offer. If the issues are beyond the group and cancer, then a referral is made in the community.

Group Agendas

In designing an ongoing, successful group, it is always important to have a structure for each session, even if you do not always get through the full agenda. Scaffolding each session based on the last is a good idea and many times group discussions may bring up new ideas or concepts that can be integrated in the next session. Keeping notes of the progress made is also a good element as well as documenting specific feelings of the group. Sometimes you might have planned to do a game, but someone had a devastating experience or doctor's visit and you have to be present with what they bring. That being said, having a format is key, but also knowing you have to be present in the moment of the group and adapt is just as important. Here is an example that is helpful to me for each session:

Tucson's Young Adult Cancer Group

Sarah F. Kurker Date: Attendees:

I. **Expectations/guidelines/collaboration**
II. **New Members Introduction**
III. **Announcements**
IV. **Update 1 thing to discuss since last group****
V. **Questions in a box**
VI. **Bright Ideas**
VII. **Post-Group Evaluation**

****If there is a new member, then we pass around an introduction sheet that the young adults came up with. Otherwise, we just give updates on what has happened since the last group.**

New Member Introduction Sheet

(please answer any or all of these questions. . . . or introduce yourself any way you like)

Name
Age
Diagnosis
Treatment
Something cool about you
Something you like
How you survived treatment
Why came to group
How has group impacted their lives?
Question for the group?

I also always have colored paper and art supplies on hand for every group
in case the young adults want to do an activity. If I do an activity that they
really liked or responded to, I keep that on hand in case we run out of things
to do. In over 4 years, I have not had that happen but it's always important
to keep the flexibility within an agenda.

Activities

Over the years, I have combined my social work skills, child life experiences and my creativity to come with formats and activities to keep the
young adults engaged during group. I do recommend trying out interventions that you think will be beneficial. You might have to change and adjust
them as you go but the best is to have a discussion with the young adults and
see what they suggest and create. I am going to highlight some of the most
successful activities that they have asked to do again and again.

Questions in A Box

Hand out pieces of paper and have everyone write a question they want
answered. It helps when there are new people since it gives them an opportunity to both learn the group and have their questions answered in a casual
and comfortable way.

I have also adapted it to be more specific if I want to lead them to a specific topic, for example, I may ask a question about body image and cancer.

Or ask a question about relationships with friends. You can start off with a broader, more generalized question and then, if they are having trouble, make it more specific. This activity is a versatile and comfortable activity that can initiate great conversations. This is one they always ask for. Often they want to do it without the box. Just in a conversation.

There are a variety of ways to "play" the game questions in a box. One way is for someone to pick a question, read and answer. I like to do this, but add the element of everyone answering it before we move on. They can answer or pass, but it elicits further discussion. Sometimes one questions can be the only discussion for that session. You can also go in order or have them pick the next person to answer. Lots of variety for one basic skill.

Free Write

Since young adults are exploring different ways to express themselves, free write is a great option since it allows the group to not only move in a more personal level but can also initiate a great discussion. First, start by introducing a theme. One example can be self-esteem. As the facilitator, you can share information about the theme, why it is relevant (I will bring a relevant article and have copies to share) as well as its significance for young adults who have gone through cancer. Then, I let them know I will be asking a flow of questions and they will just answer as they go. Then, they can share specifics of the process, or just about what they learned or not at all. They are welcome to keep their work or throw it away. The explanation on the current research or relevance is about a 5- to 10-minute summary. Then, the process of answering is about 20 to 30 minutes. Then, a discussion, but note that sometimes they don't want to discuss, it is important to be very mindful of the energy of where they are at with the end of the activity. Below are examples of a flow of questions (I like to make copies of the questions to give out so that they can take them for journaling later).

Self-Esteem Free Write Questions

What was your self-esteem prior to cancer?
How did cancer affect your self-esteem?
How have you dealt with this?
What helps you be more secure in your self-esteem?
What are you working on?
What is working?
What changes do you want to make?

Perspective Free Write Questions

What is going well in your life right now?
How does it make you feel?
How much control do you have over the good?
How does your perspective help with this?

Goal Setting Free Write Questions

What is something you have your mind on completing or accomplishing?
What steps have you taken?
What steps do you need to do?
What is in the way?
How can you get to that point?
How will your life change once you accomplish it?
How will you feel?

Appreciation Free Write Questions

Who is someone you appreciate?
What do you appreciate about them?
How has this affected you?
Have you shared it with them?
How would it make them feel?
How would it feel for you to share it?

Struggle Free Write Questions

What is something that continually bothers you?
What needs to happen for it not to bother you?
What is your part?
What do you feel about doing that?
How will it feel when this is resolved and does not bother you continually?

Once we complete them, I have them to read it over silently and ask if they want to share anything specific about what they wrote. I see if a discussion will emerge. Sometimes it's about the specifics, but sometimes about the process of the free write. As the facilitator, being patient and allowing them to share or pass is key to the success of the discussion.

Informal Group

Sometimes I will let the introductions or updates be the guide of the group. I even take the time to say tonight is your night agenda, what do you want to do or talk about. This is a free space for them to allow for leadership to emerge and guide the group to the topic that is most relevant for them at that time. It's a great change of pace and the connections that happen are really beneficial. For an ongoing group, the discussions can be draining and emotional, so allowing for connection without deep content, (unless that is what they want) is a good variation for the group process.

Bright Ideas-Problem-Solving Skills Training for Everyday Living

In the spring of 2019, I was accepted to be trained in Bright Ideas. This is an NCI evidence-based practice that has been approved and implemented across the country. The foundation of the technique is teaching patients to make their own decisions through a step-by-step process. As a social worker, you are educating them on skills that they can apply on their own. During my training, it was set up for individual support but I was able to adapt it for group purposes. I used Bright Ideas both individually and within the whole group and the young adults liked the process and ideas that Bright Ideas brought in very much.

It is important to note that some young adults may have been involved in their treatment plan and some not, depending on their age and family dynamics. Therefore, teaching bright ideas is essential to allowing them to learn the skills to plan. Many of the members of the group are faced with decisions they feel ill-equipped to make; some related to their treatment, and some as a result of all the changes to their lives. Having the tools to be able to problem solve may alleviate their distress and empower them to feel more in control of all the changes they are facing.

Social workers are trained to engage in active listening, empathy, and to enhance well-being by developing patients' and families' own skills and resources. Bright Ideas problem solving is an effective intervention in social work practice. Bright Ideas is an evidence-based cognitive behavioral intervention, which utilizes the development of constructive coping skills built around a problem-solving paradigm. It is manualized and used with parents of pediatric cancer patients as well adolescents and AYA with cancer. The "Bright" refers to the optimism that can be achieved in learning how to solve problems, and the steps are to: 1) Identify the problem, 2) Determine the best options, 3) Evaluate options, 4) Act on the options decided upon and 5) See how the solutions worked out.

Oncology social workers incorporating the Bright Ideas Intervention into their continued psychosocial support provide independence and confidence to their patients. One of the guiding principles of Bright Ideas is "Give a man a fish and feed him for a day; teach a man to fish and you feed him for a lifetime." Bright Ideas can be used in individual and group settings. The intervention has a readily available package of information and resources for clinicians and families. The creators of Bright Ideas have made all of the information and resources public and supported. Please refer to the website in the references list to review.

www.childrensoncologygroup.org/index.php/bright-ideas

Utilizing the concepts in bright ideas in the young adult group is such a benefit of the group. Since I just implemented it a year ago, I have some recommendations. One way to present it is to share the information and process. You can also get copies of the handouts and supplies for free and give to the group. The three ways I have completed it in a group are:

1. Use when only one young adult attends or if they are meeting with me alone for additional support.
2. Hand out to the whole group. Present the ideas then hand out the forms. Have then entire group work on their own sheets but it's a collective "problem." It becomes a group solving theme around Bright Ideas.
3. The most well received has been in the group setting. Each young adult gets their own paperwork and works on their own individualized issues. They have the option to share the process or keep individualized. In this role, the facilitator really needs to guide and support the process as a whole process of Bright Ideas and not their individual process.

Art Projects

We have done some artwork as a project. We create inspirational flags on fabric, and everyone puts their favorite quote in a different colored fabric pen. And then, each person takes it home. We have also done this with cards and or other art mediums. The nice part of this is they have something from their group friends to take with them, as reminders of what they learn in group.

Games

The young adults really enjoy playing games in group. We do this after check in. I usually keep games in my bag in case the discussion wanes and time is left. There are a multitude of card game questions for teens and young adults, and journals that ask about life issues. Here are some questions collected from various sources that I have compiled together.

- What person comes to mind when you hear the word, "hero" and why?
- Top 10 role models growing up? People in your life, fictional, cultural? What qualities did you admire in them?
- Discuss how you learned giving to others?
- What is role playing in social circle?
- Favorite book as teenagers and why?
- The adult who influenced me the most was.
- Important conversation with parents that showed your relationship?
- First time you stood up for yourself?
- A dream you have.
- Best advice received?
- Top 10 things you got excited or pumped about?
- Introvert or extrovert?
- Who do you connect with?
- Your relationship with nature?
- Relationship to self?

I also collect questions that the young adults have already created and make that into a game. That is the most beneficial. Below is a list of questions they have already asked.

- Is there a side effect that is still affecting your daily life?
- What did you realize that you took most for granted when you were diagnosed?
- Hardest part of how your body changed?
- How has it affected your relationships?
- How do you cope with your illness outside of group?
- What have you learned from having cancer?
- How have your life goals changed or if they haven't what are they?
- How has your diagnosis changed your outlook on things/life?

- Biggest challenge in the past week?
- What is your most helpful coping mechanism when life gets tough?
- What has your perspective on life changed since cancer?
- Do you ever feel overwhelmed with all these medical things and what do you do about it?
- Favorite thing to do during chemo in order to kill time?
- What are your goals for this year?
- How do you feel toward on how to handle stress and not knowing what to do with your free time?
- What is one great and bad thing that came out of being diagnosed with cancer?
- What was your favorite high school even that you attended or wanted to go to?
- How many pets do you have?
- When you look around and school peers are all younger then do you ever feel jealous?

Take Homes

The young adults like to work on these hard issues outside of group. I have gotten in the habit of making copies of little journal questions and or discussion questions. The young adults have used them as a visualization and also put up on their mirrors or cars! They like to take them with them at the end of group. Below are some ideas of ones I have created.

What is a perfect day for you?
What part of the day is your favorite?
How can you make this a part of this in your everyday?
What will you start doing daily to make yourself happy?

- List six things that make you happy
- How does your body feel when you are happy?
- What thoughts do you think when you are happy?
- Do you ever think of these happy things when you are sad or mad?
- How could you use these happy times?

What do you feel when you think about holidays?
What is a holiday memory that makes you happy?
How do you deal with holiday stress?
What is stress like for you?
How will you care of yourself in the holidays?

Group as a Community

Because this group is the only one in our regional area, I knew it was beneficial to provide a community for our members. The group serves as a support to those members in a multitude of ways, the biggest being connection. The young adults know they can turn to the facilitator or group members for support anytime. They can also reach out in a variety of ways to get that support. Always adding new dimensions to the group adds a dynamic that keeps them engaged in a way they are comfortable with individually. Discussed below are some significant additions to the group that were applied.

Closed Facebook Page

The closed Facebook page is only seen by members that want to join. It is a collection of regional, national and virtual events. The resources are from all over the country. I also include financial opportunities. Some of the young adults have applied and received grants for medical expenses as well as educational assistance. This has allowed for collaboration with the hospital social worker who asks me to share some of these resources for her patients.

The page also includes young adult podcast and themed programs from across the country. These have been watched and received well. It inspires them to watch young adults from other areas of the country. We have also "copied" some of the questions and themes in our group.

I also post nature photographs and or relevant quotes. It lets the young adult members know that I am there and thinking of them. They can also reach out to other members and post a question or connect outside of the group.

Another interesting thing is some young adults that have been regulars in the group, but do not attend, still want to stay on the page. It's a community even if they are not actively involved.

I also send them photographs of things we have done and announcements about upcoming group sessions or fun events. If the young adults do something together, like workout or go on a hike, or volunteer at a local program, they will post on the group. It's a safe way to stay connected.

Email or Text Communication

Having the young adults' consent to sharing their email (first 2 years of the group) and now text, is another way to connect. I usually sent a group text the day before group as a reminder. It was also beneficial in that if a young adult needed some extra support I could send them a personal text checking in. I can also give them referrals over text. Young adults often "lose" track of time so that has been a great reminder for them. I have offered to use apps like, *remind me*, but they have said they do not want to do this. With that being said, this might be a good option for other groups who may not want to use texts or emails.

Additional Private Support

Some of the young adults have had some additional psychosocial issues that they have come to me about. It may or may not be about the cancer. When I saw a pattern, I met with the funders who then allowed for me to meet with them for individual "support." It's usually before or after group session and short term, about six meetings. We utilize the Bright Ideas concept or just talk. It is offered and reminded to all young adults. Some are reluctant to see other counselors and feel comfortable because of the established relationship we have. Issues that have been needed:

1. Grief over losing a parent to cancer
2. Anxiety
3. Family issues
4. Therapy referrals
5. Relationship couples (we have a couple in our group)

Fun Events as a Young Adult Group

The young adults have really established lasting friendships outside of the group. With the financial support of Courtney's Courage (the local non-profit), our group has done some really fun "nights" off. It is always interesting to me that they do not want these events to replace the group. So, they are always in addition to. Usually, the Courtney's Courage founder and I meet them at the destination, get them the vouchers or payment and then let them have fun together. There is no financial obligation to the group members so everyone is included. Those events have been:

• Video Game and amusement mini park
• Dinners out at restaurants

- Starbucks meet ups
- Local mini golf
- Go cart racing

Other events, such as paintball and holiday events include the entire group and the leader of Courtney's Courage and myself. As requested by the young adults, we usually have a holiday party with group. We have a longer group because they still want to do the "group" with the party. It's usually a meal together, a dress up for a special event (ugly sweater, PJ or cool socks) and a card and gift card from Courtney's Courage. They have asked Kathy (From Courtney's Challenge), to share about her foundation and her daughter too.

These additional "fun" activities serve a multitude of benefits for the young adults. It gives them a break from the challenging things we discuss in group. It gives them an opportunity to establish stronger relationships, be part of a social interaction, which after cancer, some are not. It also allows for them to practice social skills during the events. This past year they have asked to do it about four times a month and they ask for particular events that all are welcome to do. They are very aware of events that would defer some from attending and they do not pick those.

Volunteering

The group transitioned to the Ronald McDonald House of Southern Arizona, 2 years back. There are multiple advantages of having it there. The first reason was no one who was admitted was feeling well enough to attend. The ones that did come to group didn't have physical or emotional adverse feelings to be back on the unit where they had a lot o trauma. It changed the atmosphere of the group into a more comfortable and surviving group. The Ronald McDonald House (RMDH) always welcomes us to eat the meals prepared by community volunteers, so we have the feeling of being out. Then, we go into their private room to do our group. It's a comfortable nice setting without the medical disturbances. It has also been beneficial since a lot of patients stay there and can attend after treatments. Many of the ongoing young adults give back by making a meal for RMDH with their families to give back. It usually is an event of when they finished treatment.

The young adults as a group volunteer at the Candelighter's annual prom. They go as a group and help others (and have fun together at the same time). It's the prom they attended while they were in treatment. They have also volunteered at Candelighters camps for patients and siblings.

As mentioned before, many of the young adults have been in Courtney's courage annual events as speakers. They share about their experience and how the group has affected them.

Coronavirus

In March of 2020, the global pandemic affected our group. Fortunately, our group had been utilizing Zoom for the past year for those adults that's immune system was so low that they could not attend. So, we quickly just changed our meetings over to Zoom. It is different but the connection was still there. Also, the young adults were able to privately answer the pre- and post-evaluation over the chat feature. They asked for some additional Zooms for some psychoeducation, such as meditation, stretch and yoga. They were in addition to group and shorter in time. The young adults were able to ask for what they need in trying times. The virus triggered a lot for most of them. Many of them had had bone marrow transplants, where they were isolated for months at a time. So, it brought that and the use of masks back. Life stopped like it did when they were going through cancer treatments so group was more important than ever to help with some of those triggers.

Always There

The importance of this group was reinforced when I received a text from a young adult who attended the group years ago, for about five sessions. I had not heard from him for about a year yet he reached out to me to share that he was feeling down. We exchanged texts and I helped him. I gave him a quote that I thought was relevant to his issues and then told him about upcoming groups. The power of this connection is strong—who would he have turned to if not connected to the group? There is great satisfaction in helping this underserved population, young adults with cancer. It helps me to be a better social worker and faculty instructor and that connection enlightens me.

4 Pre- and Post-Evaluation Significance of Group Support Structures

Introduction

Evaluation is an important component to the success of a young adult cancer support group. Consistently asking for feedback from the group allows for greater participation. Evaluations also validate that not only are members benefiting from the group but they are also providing valuable information to help other young adults going through cancer. The significance of their experience and young adults' participation in giving back is a key component to the process of evaluating the dynamics within a group. The gift of giving back; post-traumatic growth, fuels young adults to be active and take ownership of the group, and allows them an outlet to provide support to others from their experience. As a social worker, this connection of the group as a community allows young adults to take control of their own healing, generating many therapeutic entities. I always admire how anytime they are asked to give ideas about group formatting it gives meaning to their cancer experience, providing something positive from the challenge. This is a core social work value, listening to the clients and letting them be a part of their healing. By the young adults integrating their experiences to help others, it gives them a sense of purpose and control that they may have lost during cancer. Therefore, especially in a young adult group, evaluation has a therapeutic significance to the healing of the participants.

Developmentally young adults are trying to identify who they are independently from their family of origin. Because of the demands of cancer treatment, young adults often are challenged by this because of the nature of becoming more dependent on their parents or caregivers as they go through treatment. Therefore, it is a secondary challenge for young adults to navigate their personal identity development. While losing control of choices, surviving the physical effects of treatment and becoming more dependent in a time when they should be less dependent on their family is a key component of group. Because of this, it should be noted that "knowledge sharing and communications are needed throughout the transition from cancer care into community care. AYA survivors are likely to need developmentally appropriate psychosocial care as well and extensive follow-on surveillance" (Dahlke, Fair, Hong, Kellsedt, & Ory, 2017). Being aware, as a clinical social worker, of what each young adult can address in the moment is key to proving the most effective support. Some young adults deal with and process these issues positively during treatment while others are unable to process till after because they are in survival mode. Balancing what the young adults and the group can handle is a skill that the facilitator constantly processes. The therapeutic work that can be accomplished individually and within a group demands constant reflection by the facilitator. Evaluation can be a tool to help social work facilitators with this process.

During the past 3 years of bimonthly support groups, I have created and revised many evaluations. The examples in this chapter are following for clinicians to utilize. Based on social work research, the use of Likert scales and open-ended questions are valuable to evaluate programs. I have combined and changed many of these as I have moved through and gained experience with the developing group. Depending on the demographics of the region of your support group and the actual design of the group, you will be able to formulate the best evaluation for you (Feel free to utilize the actual examples). Below each evaluation, I have attached both the strengths and weaknesses of each modality. It is suggested to change up your evaluations at least every 6 months. This evaluative change for the young adults keeps them engaged and challenged in their responses. From my experience, once you notice shorter answers and feedback, this is a good indication that it's time to adjust the evaluation.

When thinking about which survey to use or combination of the following piloted evaluations you would like to use, consider having some type of scale and open-ended questions. This purpose is twofold. First, young adults may choose to answer only one type of question. That way you are giving them the option and allowing for information to be gathered. It also gives them some control in the information they are wanting to share. Another key component to combining them is to have both qualitative and quantitative. As a clinical social worker, it is our obligation to give back to the profession of social work. The more information you have, the more you can share. You may present this information at a conference or be a field supervisor to a student and having this valuable information is always a tool that validates the efficacy of the work. Because there is not a lot of data and research on how to facilitate a young adult group with cancer, you will be contributing to the profession by collecting it. You will also be allowing the young adults to have a voice, giving them strength and power through personal empowerment. In some cases, agencies or funding services ask for evaluations. "The development of survivorship research methods and measurable outcomes to support evidence-based educational materials and guidelines depend of the availability of funding opportunities" (Dahlke et al., 2017). Thus, evaluations are a way to ensure the funding and continuation of group. An evaluation can be shared to funders and give them an idea of the impact the group has on young adults with cancer in their lives. Therefore, evaluations are critical to providing effective social work interventions on any level.

Limitations of the Group Evaluations

Looking at the research on support groups, and then reviewing the possible evaluations I have utilized, I see some issues that are lacking. I have never considered asking the young adults about the support their parents receive. Offering support sessions for young adults and their families would be valuable. If the group facilitator is unable to provide, this a referral to someone in the community that can be appropriate. Something as simple as conducting a seminar in which the young adults can invite their parents to provide both support and communication which would benefit the relationships between them and their parents. "It is necessary to help and support the parents in order to help and support the children" (Landry-Dattée et al., 2016). There are just so many dynamics that professionals can contribute to. It also makes sense since most research will only fund if it's a multi-centered collaboration. It is in reflection like this that I see the significance as I review my work and how it compares to current research.

Another component that the group evaluation does not ask about is the online closed Facebook community. This social media platform needs to be included in the evaluation. "Face-to-face support groups may facilitate more sense-making of past events through storytelling and positive feedback and that online support groups may be better provide space to express negative feelings, engage in information seeking for decision-making and discuss sensitive topics like friendships and sex" (Thompson, Crook, Love, Macpherson, & Johnson, 2016). Because the Candlelighters group is face-to-face and online, it would be valuable to allow the young adults to give feedback on both platforms.

Evaluation Options

Example 1

This evaluation was developed by some of the young adults who have attended my groups. They liked formulating the feeling circles, similar to the pain scale they do in the clinic. From a social work perspective, this evaluation tool is one that would leave a lot unanswered unless you are more directive in asking them to answer additional follow-up questions.

> (this example would be smaller and to scale of the page for review (full copies in appendixes)
> Pre-Group:
> I feel: (circle)

1. Write one word that explains how you have been feeling this past week?
2. What is one thing that has been heavy on your mind?
3. What do you want to talk about in group today?

> Other comments you want to share?
> Post-Group:
> I feel: (circle)

1. Name a color you feel you are now that group is over? How about a word?
2. What is one thing that you felt group helped you with today?
3. What is something you would like to discuss in our next group?

Other comments you want to share:

Example 2

This was the first evaluation I created. I wanted to have an evaluative tool that had open-ended questions and a scale. I also wanted it to be simple and fast, seeing as we were just creating the group. The advantage of this one, or a simple one like it, is that you can get at the content you really want to evaluate quickly. In addition, it takes less time for them to complete and is focused about what you want to find out. With a quick survey, you always want to leave a space for anything they want to share. If it is just multiple choice or a Likert scale, then young adults don't have the opportunity to share something that is concerning to them or an issue they want to bring up. If you utilize this option, it can be easily adjusted to evaluate certain themes you want to assess.

How I feel emotionally before group:

> (please circle)
> Bad 1.....2.....3.....4.....5.....6.....7.....8.....9.....10 Good
> Comments:
> What would you like to discuss in group?
> Post-Group

How I feel emotionally after group:

(please circle)
Bad 1.....2.....3.....4.....5.....6.....7.....8.....9.....10 Good
Suggestions for the group:
What I liked:
What I did not like:

Example 3

This group evaluation is another brief and direct survey that focuses on the emotions that the young adults are feeling. You can swap out the emotions or add to this evaluation depending on what you are wanting to assess.

Pre-Group
I feel happy_____

5	4	3	2	1
Strongly Agree	Agree	Neutral	Disagree	Strongly Disagree

Why I came to group today
Post-Group
I feel happy_____

5	4	3	2	1
Strongly Agree	Agree	Neutral	Disagree	Strongly Disagree

I feel the group helped support me today_____

5	4	3	2	1
Strongly Agree	Agree	Neutral	Disagree	Strongly Disagree

What I got out of group today
Please take some time to share how the group has impacted your life:

Example 4

I created this evaluation after consistently hearing complaints about filling out the evaluations. The young adults in my group seem to like the openness of the following evaluation because it assesses their before- and after-group perspective. For the pre, I ask them to write down *why they came to group this week*. Then, for the post, at the end of the group meeting, I ask them what they want to share with me about group or *what they got from group tonight*. Leaving it open-ended for both the pre- and post-responses on index cards has given me more variety in their responses. Sometimes they share that they need to meet alone about a personal issue or express gratitude to me for being there for them. The openness and freedom of this evaluation are effective.

> Use a blank index card.
> Pre-Group
> Why did you come to group today?
> Post-Group
> What did you gain from group today?

Group Example Discussion

These four examples have been piloted over the past 3 years. There are strengths and weaknesses in each evaluation. As long as you are consistent in utilizing them, they are effective. If you run into issues where the young adults don't want to fill them out, just remind them of the importance of their feedback in helping both the material to become more effective and the growth of the facilitator. Remind them that it also contributes to better clinical care for new patients. It gives a purpose to their cancer; their way to give back.

Each of the four examples provides the opportunity to share feedback, screen for individual issues that may not come up in group, and check to make sure of the mental well-being of your participants.

In terms of evaluating both your group and your skills as a facilitator, these evaluations are critical in proving that evidence-based interventions are beneficial. In reviewing current research for this book, most of the journals discuss that young adults are an underserved cancer population. As I reviewed my limitations on the MGH group and the Candelighter's Group, one aspect I saw was the small pilot size. While this may be perceived as a limitation, it can also be looked at as the foundation for the necessity of more research. As oncology social workers who want to provide the best evidence-based interventions, it is our ethical responsibility to contribute to research. Pilot research can be the foundation of further research. Every young adult that participates can influence a clinician or another young adult. Some research also states that social workers need to participate at any level of research and collaborate with other social workers and share their insight. There are so many clinical issues that young adults face and by participating in evidence-based research we can further comprehend the intricate issues young adults with cancer face. "Very little research has explored the role of facilitators in online communities" (Griffiths, Panteli, Brunton, Marder, & Williamson, 2015). Any data we provide as clinical social workers will contribute to more understanding. By gathering evaluations from your group, you are not only contributing to data but also evolving the topics, the flow and the communication within group.

Contributions From the Evaluations

Evaluations from Tucson's Young Adult Cancer Group: (young adults from age 16 to 25, 2017 to 2020).

> This group helps me with life's struggles and how to deal with emotions over all. It has taught me how to deal with the hard times.
> Group has impacted my life tremendously! I started going to group two months before the end of my treatment. When I started going I instantly felt welcome and support in every way I needed. When these things happen (cancer) no one can fully understand, but coming here meeting people who go through similar things and we can at least understand a little helps so much with mental health which leads the way for physical health.

Part of the group is psychoeducation. Educating the young adults about the connection between mind and body well-being is very important. They often ask about different modalities that they want to learn, meditation, gratitude journals and yoga. We discuss this link in group as it comes up with their experiences. I am also an active participant in YAG articles, podcasts and online supports. When there are relevant articles, I bring copies and summarize them in group. That way it broadens the horizon of these young adults from a small-town mentality to a more expansive outlook. It is important to summarize the information as well as hand material and resources out to them. Some young adults are invested in learning outside of the group so reaching out with verbal and written communication is profound.

> Group for me has provided an outlet for all my stress, worries, anxiety and fears that cancer has given me". It has connected me with people who have a deep understanding for similar circumstances we face. There is not a single outlet other than this group where young individuals who never experienced such trauma come together and provide support and positivity in other's life. I am eternally grateful for this support.

Allowing the young adults to express the pain they went through is so important. A lot of times I hear that they don't have anyone to share it with.

They don't want to worry their parents (or caregivers). Their friends just don't understand. And many times, these young adults feel that their in-hospital social worker (or psychosocial support person) is either there for their parents or they personally are not physically able to deal with the emotional side of treatment while being treated so they don't take advantage of that support. So, for many, this is the first time they have the opportunity and are ready to share their emotional side of their cancer. Providing a safe place for them to revisit these emotions allows for emotional healing from the cancer trauma.

> Group to me means that I have someone to support me and tell me things that give me advice about things I'm not sure about. These people mean so much to me because they don't pass away judgment. There is so much communication and development within this group that impacts me and help with all of my difficulties and trials.

A theme that I have observed in the years of facilitating this ongoing group is that on many levels, it's a social skill training group. Many of the young adults have missed out on the communication and social skills that they would have learned in school due to treatment and isolation from a social network. They missed out on important relationships that would have had them better prepared, so when they go into the "real" world after cancer, their social skills are lacking. These issues come up at every session and is a key developmental issue to address.

> This support group has impacted my life very positively. It is extremely therapeutic to me to be able to come to a safe place to share mutual feelings with people who can completely understand the traumatic experiences I went through.
>
> On rough days and when I feel hopeless, this group provides me with the strength and faith I lose sight of. I'm forever grateful to have a safe haven that is surrounded with others who share the pain and concerns that come with facing cancer. I am blessed with the opportunity to attend this group and meet other who have come from the same journey.

Creating a community is a foundational aspect of the group. Even if the young adults are too busy, in treatment or too sick to come, they still have that connection that they are not alone. They can reach out and someone will support them, providing a connection of understanding of what they are going through. They have a list of 24/7 helplines. They also can text one another or provide contact over social media. They also can communicate with the group facilitator and set up an individual meeting as needed.

Gives me a sense of purpose. Help others, see friends. Socialize.

Happy we have someone new, I hop can help her out!

Very happy to meet a new person. It's sad to hear about her suffering, but it's reassuring to know there can be an end to treatment-I just hope everything goes well. It means a lot to me to help other people. I have been thinking that even once I move out of state eventually that I would like to find a way to mentor/support AYA patient and survivors in the future.

I came for emotional support and to hear from everyone. I got support an advice and I hope I helped someone.

Post-traumatic growth is something that comes up in each group. The fact that not only are they showing up to talk about deep emotional issues, they are sharing to better help others. They are taking a chance of working on their own issues, sharing vulnerability with the hope that it may trigger support in another young adult. The risk of bonding and sharing and the experiences of relapse and death are always present. But they do it for both themselves and others. This enables them to have meaning in this time of post-treatment while not actively moving forward with traditional milestones (due to treatment restriction). It's a gateway to moving forward and recognizing the positive impact they are making on others.

I came to support other and get support myself. The pain clinic helped me figure out what is important force this group is. It's good for finding purpose in my life.

Group made me feel like I wasn't alone. That's how it helped me.

Relieves of a little stress and always good to see how everyone feels about their treatment or life obstacles.

I like that more people are showing up.

Really helped me sort through old memories and taught me good coping skills.

Motivated me to do good. Thanks for the motivation to keep improving and new ways to relieve stress.

I want to learn meditation.

I'd like to know how to manage more than one thing at a time.

It is the responsibility of the facilitator to not just read but understand the implications of these evaluations are saying. Often times when asked, the young adults might not feel comfortable expressing what they want in the group. By having them continuously evaluate the group, they are able to eventually express what they might be looking for. Many times, they want to learn about yoga or meditation, so allowing for education and resources in the group brings a level of empowerment to different modalities of healing. If your community treatment center provides alternative therapies, you can invite collaborative psycho-oncology practitioners to attend group and give brief psychoeducation on what they provide. Often times, young adults have misinformation about what this means and after being educated, they are more open to trying supportive care. Not only does this benefit your young adults but it also provides a networked means of communication in your community to provide the best care for young adults. Part of providing a group out of this group, community referrals are vital to providing comprehensive care.

References

Dahlke, D., Fair, K., Hong, Y., Kellsedt, D., & Ory, M. (2017). Adolescent and young adult cancer survivorship educational programming: A qualitative evaluation. *JMIR Cancer, 3*(1), e3.

Griffiths, C., Panteli, N., Brunton, D., Marder, B., & Williamson, H. (2015). Designing and evaluating the acceptability of realshare: An online support community for teenagers and young adults with cancer. *Journal of Health Psychology, 20*(12), 1589–1601.

Landry-Dattée, N., Boinon, D., Roig, G., Bouregba, A., Delaigue-Cosset, M.-F., & Dauchy, S. (2016). Telling the truth . . . with kindness: Retrospective evaluation of 12 years of activity of a support group for children and their parents with cancer. *Cancer Nursing, 39*(2), E10–E18.

Thompson, C. M., Crook, B., Love, B., Macpherson, C. F., & Johnson, R. (2016). Understanding how adolescents and young adults with cancer talk about needs in online and face-to-face support groups. *Journal of Health Psychology, 21*(11), 2636–2646.

5 Life Lessons From the Young Adults

Thank you. I am excited for the future and know after tonight's talk everything will be okay. Thank you for always proving Hope!

Chapter Overview

This entire chapter is dedicated to the young adult participants in Tucson, Arizona over the past 4 years. It exemplifies their experience in being a member of the support group and community connection. Their honest and consistent participation in the evolving evaluations are the foundation of relevant themes. These themes identified the needs of young adults with cancer. Allow these to be the foundation of themes you begin to address in your support group. They will elicit more discussion and themes that are prevalent in the young adult's lives. Another benefit to their thoughts is to use this as an activity to promote discussion about the themes in your groups.

Focus

The focus of this chapter is to present the collection of feedback from our group. The themes are categorized, and then, there is clinical feedback for each. These clinical observations connect the issues discussed in each chapter of the book. The main purpose of presenting this data is to incorporate the psychosocial needs of young adults in a community group setting.

Aims

The aim of this chapter is to present the feedback to inspire support groups addressing these physical and emotional developmental issues. These sections provide valuable ideas for clinicians to more fully evaluate their existing support groups for young adults, and creating new ones that fit the needs of your community.

Evaluations Summary

For the past 4 years of the Tucson Community Support Group, the young adults have provided significant evaluation responses that have helped shape both the structure and direction of the group. The following feedback is intended to help in the formulation of your specific group. It should also provide insight to social workers in evaluating the ongoing needs of young adult cancer survivors. Each insight can be a basis for a group theme or concept to develop in a group.

The combination of feedback comes from the various evaluations presented in Chapter 4. The data from these evaluations have been synthesized them into working themes for clinicians. The themes identify the major concerns of young adults facing cancer. Some fall into the developmental stages presented in Chapter 1, specifically, physical, emotional dimensions. There are some new elements identified under the emotional component which are significant to address in group.

The collection of data from the community support groups are presented in this chapter; they are listed under each theme and appear in italics. They are structured together, and my clinical observations are presented thereafter. This chapter provides a road map for supportive and fruitful discussions in support groups with young adults with cancer.

Community

Group was good and got to talk a lot.
Good talk about my experiences.
I love everything about group
It's a good place to just hang out.
They made me come to group, so I thought I'd give it a try.
I hadn't been to group in a while and I really wanted to go.
I'm here to meet some cool people.
I liked tonight and getting to talk and see and hear from everyone.
I will definitely come again!
See friends, support, fun, meeting new people.
Group was fun, always good to have new people.

Support socialization, entertainment.
Because there was group.
To see everyone.
I really liked getting to know everyone.
I came to group today because my boyfriend thought it would be heal-
ing for me.
I am glad I went to group tonight.
Just thought I would come.
I came to group this week cause I thought the last group went well and
wanted to continue and learn more.
Have been a while and wanted to catch up.
Because I love to come to group I love it!!
I came to group to see and talk to J. and K.
I came to group to celebrate Christmas with group.
Came to group to check in with group mates.
I came because I haven't been to group in a while & felt it would be
helpful to come.

The main objective of this book is that a young adult oncology support group is the foundation of a community for this underserved population. Because their needs are so unique at this developmental age, building a community for them helps them in countless ways. The community allows them to feel connected and safe. Because issues constantly come up from surviving cancer, they have a stable place to share openly, without the fear of worrying their loved ones. This community also allows the young adults to explore their identity and share their process of finding themselves after surviving cancer.

When reviewing their words, this community provides well beyond a safe support for them, it is always there, and provides these young adults with consistency of support. As reflected by their comments, some have not attended for a while but are always welcome. Having a safe place to not worry about other's reactions is part of the foundation of this community. And unlike professional help; just by surviving cancer, there is a mutual understanding of their feelings, identities and experiences. As the facilitator witnessing this connection, it is profound and something only a young adult cancer support community can provide.

With that being said, there is also heartbreak by joining a group like this. The reality is that some of our members have died. And facing death in this community brings about a lot of emotions for all. When we have had members that have died, we come together as a group to honor and respect that member. At the same time, we acknowledge what that does to our members, bringing fear of the unknown to the forefront of our group discussions. As these young adults have faced this since their diagnosis, they come together to acknowledge that it's there.

Validation of Cancer Experience

The group was amazing; it was really helpful . . . to meet people who have experienced the same things I have.

It was nice and not half bad. I learned a lot about different people with cancer.

I came to group because I just wanted to get a break from crazy business of end of cancer stuff. This gives me an extra space to relax.

Being more comfortable with scars.

I liked group tonight because it is therapeutic to talk about similar traumas with other people who can relate while feeling comfortable in a safe environment.

I came to group tonight because I'm trying to cope with my traumas.

Support laughs sharing medial experiences. Mental preparing for potential surgeries.

It was helpful hearing other people's perspectives on coping and their traumas that were just as similar as they were different.

I came to group tonight to heal and relate to other people who had been through similar traumas as me.

This is my first time coming to group. I came to group because after what I went through my family choose to forget about it so I wanted to see what it felt like to talk about my experience.

Very happy to meet a new person. It's sad to hear about her suffering, but its reassuring to know there can be an end to treatment. I just hope everything goes well. It means a lot to me to help other people.

After three plus years of dealing with my illness, I decided that it could be good for me to attend this meeting.

It was nice begin able to share my feelings about my traumas in a safe environment with people who had similar experiences.

Meet new people. Reflect on two years since surgery for testicular cancer.

I came because I've been feeling super frustrated about the surgery and G. feels like taking 1 step forward and 100 back.

I came to group because I hadn't been to group in around a month and I was feeling like I needed a little more support since my last chemo.

Just to come.

Met a new person.

I came to see everyone! I loved seeing everyone and hearing from everyone.

Wanted to meet others.

As an oncology social worker, there was no evidence-based practice intervention that would provide the validation of what really happened being diagnosed and treated for cancer, especially for young adults. Everything I learned was from a young adult's personal experience. And what I found was getting them together in a clinical setting, the flow of validation happens. No matter the young adult's socio-economic background, or cultural identity, they can bond and support like this connection. Often my social work "advice" to one patient was from another patient in the next room. They just got it. That is why a young adult support group is so valuable to their healing.

As seen in their evaluations, the validation of their cancer experience is very important in their healing and moving on from cancer. Being able to openly evaluate things that have happened to them on a physical and emotional level is important in their process of moving on. In comparison to individual therapy, the group share is something so profound that it allows them to move forward with an understanding from others who have been through it. Being able to voice their experience and understanding to a group who has gone through it is invaluable. They seem to really be able to see a new perspective to their experience when others share.

As mentioned throughout this book, being able to freely share, without judgment or the worry of stressing out loved ones, this group allows for the expression of sometimes unshared feelings. This is so significant to moving forward in their new identity. They are able to grieve their past precancer selves and visions. They are able to really **feel** without overloading their loved ones. I often hear that they feel guilty to share these experiences with their loved ones as they have already caused them so much heartache in seeing them suffer. This is uniquely important to the experience of a young adult.

Being Heard

> *I need it to talk.*
> *Ability to express myself.*
> *I got support and advice and I hope I helped someone.*
> *Talking about what hanging over my mind.*
> *I got the support I needed and the advice I think I needed.*
> *What I got out of group was . . . I finally met J and got to hear a bit about her story. I also got updates on M and E.*
> *It was great to catch up with everyone and share good thoughts with one another. Praying and missing G.*

Over the past few years, I have learned that while in treatment some young adults are not able to share their feelings. They are on survival mode, literally, and it's too difficult to address. With the developmental age to be more independent, they also are reluctant to go to the support of a professional. They don't want to share with loved ones as to protect them. So just having a safe place to be heard is part of the needed benefit of a young adult cancer support group.

As oncology social workers and other oncology professionals, we quickly learn that the cancer experience does not have a "cure." It's life-changing and constantly impacting our patients. Allowing them to just be heard is therapeutic. In being heard and sharing their experiences, they are able to come to a greater understanding within the process of sharing. Being heard is particularly important to this experience and provides a deeper understanding and ability for them to cope.

Support Group Suggestions

Really like the activity and book reading.
I still really like the questions.
Not enough people
I like the free style of topics of today's group.
I came to group because I hadn't been in a while and had a lot going on lately and felt I would need support.
I enjoyed the questions that we were able to discuss out loud. We should do those more often.
Remember when to go.
Maybe write something you feel or that bugs you, and you like rip it up to help you kind of let it go.
Tonight's group was really good! Liked pretty much everything.
I really like the questions.
Today's group was fun, I liked the questions.
Healthy snacks for veggies and fruit.
I like having open and conversations rather than questions in a box.
Love the honesty, need more people for some activities.
More questions, I love the questions.
More open discussion, good time.
Social worker recommended this two July's ago. Was surgery for testicular cancer.
Right amount of time.
The topics were good.
Open discussion portion.

Chapter 4 is dedicated to the importance of evaluation in creating the most relevant and helpful support group community. Part of the importance of evaluation is to give the young adults a voice in the structure of their group. As noted in their responses, they have creative and constructive suggestions for the group. Incorporating their suggestions gives them a voice in the group and more dedication to attending if they know their opinion counts.

Meaning/Identity

> *I came to support others and get support myself. The pain clinic helped me figure out what is important for me and this group is. This is good for finding purpose in my life.*
>
> *I got to list the changes in my life and it motivated me to try to solve these issues in my life.*
>
> *I come to group to get out of the house. Didn't have plans all day.*
>
> *Give me some sense of purpose. Help other. See friends. Happy we have someone new, hope I can help her out!*

The community support group gives some young adults a purpose. Many have stopped school and are unable to work. Life is on hold and attending the group gives them a reason to look forward. When recovering from treatment, young adults are working on their new identity after cancer. But it's hard to work on these issues without being involved in some outside connection. The participation can be the first step to find more meaning and direction in their lives.

Connectedness

> *Helps keep connected.*
>
> *Today I got traditions from everyone and felt closer than I would if I hadn't known these thing.*
>
> *It's being a while that I've talked to teens and people that I can actually relate to*
>
> *I came to group to interact and just get out of the house.*
>
> *I am here tonight to make some positive connections and get some real life interaction.*
>
> *I came to group because I hadn't left the house and I felt I needed to stimulate my mind a little and talk to group mates.*
>
> *I feel so much love and understanding from their group. I feel relieved and content with opening. Thankful for all the great advice.*
>
> *Hearing how everyone is doing.*
>
> *It was nice hearing from H. and her experiences b/c I could relate to many of her stories.*
>
> *Group made me feel like I wasn't alone. That how it helped me.*

Coming to group helped me so much hearing other people's stories.

I enjoyed hearing the new group members' stories because they related to my story. It was nice hearing they had similar issues as me and it was a relief to know that there are others going through the same thing as me.

Group was great and I love how everyone connected and how healing.

I came because this is a very hard thing to go through and sometimes it feels like no one gets it.

It's a sense of relief to know I'm not the only one going through this. Felt comfortable sharing my experience with the group.

I like the people.

Tonight I thought group was good and its nice to know/meet other people and what they had and their stories.

Ask each person if had similar experience.

It's nice to just talk to other teens.

Support, social.

Made me feel like I'm not the only one.

The relations that can be made here.

I came to group to feel understood.

This is one of the most valuable parts of the community support group—connection. Feeling connected is the foundation of their needs. These feeling of connection is a really significant part of being a member of the group. This feeling also allows for deeper conversations within the group. Once these young adults feel this connection, they share deeper issues within the group.

With young adults, once they feel this connection, their confidence and ability to share increases exponentially. They are more willing to try new techniques and get out of their comfort zone in group sessions.

This also flows into their relationships outside of the group. They are able to work on other parts of their lives such as working on family dynamics. Oftentimes, cancer causes additional friction between siblings. Sometimes the work within relationships actually occurs in group, with feedback from their peers. In some cases, the work only needs to happen in their group. It is more a realization of the perspective that they need to hear and see.

Coping Skills

I had so much fun and need to work on coping mechanism.

To talk and relief stress.

I'm here because I wanted to interact with my friends.

Relieve stress, talk.

> *I learned that we all have problems in life and we all cope with them in different ways.*
> *I came to see everyone and to get the support I needed.*
> *Tonight I feel as I am leaving with a clear mind and a better version of myself.*
> *Really helped me sort through old memories and taught me good coping skills.*
> *Friends, opportunity for support and to support others. Socializing.*
> *I came to the group for some quality social interaction.*

Coping skills are vital to living a positive life. Many young adults missed the opportunity to practice coping skills during their transition to adulthood. Since they were focused on treatment and survival, they missed those opportunities. There is also the component of the continued dependence upon their parents. Because of their diagnosis and treatment, young adults rely heavily on their parents and other family caregivers. The boundaries between the young adults and their caregivers/parents become blurred, and the transition back to independence is difficult for these young adults since they need practice on their coping skills. This group allows them to practice and learn these skills so they can utilize them as they grow into their adult life.

Psychosocial Education

> *Group was good we answered good questions.*
> *Had my questions answered.*
> *Have a specific topic medication.*
> *The intro name diagnoses and everyone ask them a question*
> *Yoga*
> *I want to learn meditation.*
> *I would like to know how to manage more than one thing at a time.*
> *I learned that "migraine therapy" is a thing.*

Support groups are an ideal platform to learn about specific skills and interventions. Once the young adults are comfortable within the group, they feel empowered to seek help as to particular needs they are facing. Support groups are an invaluable means to introduce different therapies and skills to young adults. Once they experience the benefits of such support over time, they actively seek out additional support and guidance from their facilitator and the community.

In advance of each group session, information on primary issues facing young adults should be organized for prestation to the group, and a lesson, activity and follow-up on coping skills should be honed through the continuing sessions. That ensures they are able to balance their new skills and try them out in "real" life. Written materials and resource references should be provided at each session such that our young adults have these resources at their disposal whenever needed.

Perspective

> *To take everyone's comment into consideration.*
> *Hearing others ideas and what they are up to.*
> *It was nice to hear everyone and have perspective validated.*
> *Like the other peoples input.*
> *I am not good at suggestions! Helped get a better perspective. I give up easily because not sure what I want in life.*
> *Heard other people's point of view.*
> *It felt great to talk and listen to someone else going through something similar although very different.*
> *I came to group to see and hear from others.*
> *This was a pretty neat experience. I appreciate getting to hear someone else perspective.*

The foundation of success of group for this underserved population is learning new perspectives from peers. In every session, every activity these young adults are exposed to present new angles to the experiences they had. This gives them great depth as to issues they present within the group.

The balance of learning from their peers in group and then getting clinical guidance from the facilitator is a huge benefit. The young adults that become bonded with their facilitator can also meet with them individually if specific issues come up. Sometimes if there is a persistent issue that a facilitator observes, they can meet with the young adult individually to address those issues. Often, the young adult comes to the facilitator for extra support. This can enhance the group overall with the additional and individualized support.

Communication Skills

> *Talking about what bothers me in my life helps letting go of guilt for having a different bond with my mom.*
> *I liked everyone being open.*
> *I enjoyed the meetup. I find the social interaction beneficial.*
> *I came to group to see everyone.*
> *I like that more people are showing up.*

Communication skills are always being practiced in group. Since the young adults are not fully back into society, just attending group helps with language skills. This is a great practice and always with each session then it increases their confidence. The level of communication is underlined with confidence. Most young adults who have survived cancer have some level of fear to meet new people. This is the opportunity to discuss it as well as practice in group.

Life Skills

Stressed about how to talk about cancer to others.

Feel relief of a little stress and always good to see how everyone feels about their treatments or life obstacles.

I revisited that I need to take it day by day as I recover.

I really found the bright ideas activity insanely helpful. It added some reassurance to some problems that I am facing and how I could go about solving them.

Before- Good spirits. Realizing how my attitude affects me and others.

Feeling much better relived to talk about my mom and issues I am having.

Came because I have been reflecting on this last year and personal growth. I have had a lot to do with the communication that happens in group.

This was a good night. I feel that the discussion was productive and directly addressed the problems that I have been hugely negatively affecting me. There were actionable steps being provided, and my #1 takeaways was how important it is to be present, rather than in my own head.

I think my biggest take away is that I need to block out time for just enjoying things without analyzing. I need to relax more and just take it easy. All in all, we are all our own spin doctors and we control our own narrating.

Because I wanted to speak to some about my life events.

I came to group because I am looking to be in a good place

Life skills are the ways to succeed and be flexible from day to day. In group, members talk about how they handle life issues and stress. They are also able to process feedback from their peers. This process of gaining life skills by participating in the group is invaluable to young adults that have missed normal opportunities to practice these skills as their life has been on hold during cancer treatment.

Participants talk about the vast array of experiences they have encountered since they joined the support group, and they share how they navigated those issues. The others recommend how to respond, and or how they responded in similar situation. By confiding in the group about life experiences, it enables them to get feedback and ideas on these situations that they may have missed out on.

Sometimes in group, the facilitator will present different life "role play" activities. The young adults really like this as they can practice these life skills in a safe environment. Then, they can practice these skills in the outside world and get feedback on their experiences in the upcoming group.

Mental Health

Wanted to meet other cancer patients and my mental health sucks.

I came to group because I felt like my depression might have been getting bad and I needed a positive outlet.

After thinking on stories, stresses out and back on depression pills.

Talked about some irrational fears.

I feel so much better & got a lot of help involving my therapy and personal issues.

I came to group because I think it is helpful for my mental health.

I came to group because I had high anxiety today and I thought group could help.

I'm here because as I've been thinking, I'm starting to realize just how much my physical health has been affecting me,

and how my mental health has been affecting my physical health.

I came to group because I felt defeated and overwhelmed.

Because it mentally helps me retract myself in how to cope with the next month.

Mood changes needed positivity.

Had a panic attack about relapsing earlier this week.

Many young adults have faced some type of trauma pertaining to their mental health. Some have had some ups and downs in life and some have had a diagnosis of mental illness prior to cancer. Some have had challenging childhoods and experienced "a tough life." The commonality I have seen is that going through cancer treatment exacerbates the preexisting mental health struggles.

For the young adults that have not had a diagnosis, or any type of struggle, depression and anxiety become prevalent during and after treatment. Many times this is the "push" that gets them to support group. They state they have been feeling sad or lonely and it brings them to group.

Therefore, discussing mental illness and ways to get support through it is very significant. For some, just being able to share they have these feelings is helpful. Other members need to be referred to therapists and or doctors for support.

A big discussion in group is the balance of these mental illnesses due to the experience or side effect of a medication they are on. Sharing this side effect is important to see what other's experienced and how they shared it with their oncology team to address.

Emotional Outlet

> *Thank you, like today I felt like shit when I walk in. Now I feel better.*
> *I got to talk about things.*
> *Got a lot of stress out.*
> *I came for emotional support and to hear from everyone.*
> *All good.*
> *1 on 1 talk.*
> *Tonight I came because recovery has been difficult and having a (+) mindset.*
> *Feel better about progress and how slow and its fine to feel frustrated.*
> *It felt to distress after a long week.*
> *Still in a holding pattern trying to figure out what comes next.*
> *I feel relieved my & my heart feels lighter and sorry for being so emotional.*
> *Feel a lot calmer knowing I am not alone in the issues I am feeling.*
> *Being able to talk to other people about shared experiences was great and helped me go on a path of healing.*

What I have heard over the years as an oncology social worker is that this population feels a lot of guilt about how cancer has affected their lives. They are very cognizant that their parents worry about them. They know that as a parent, watching their child fight for their life is extremely painful. They know siblings get neglected. They feel the disconnect that happens within their family and they want to protect their loved ones from their emotions.

The support group allows them to feel whatever they feel about their cancer experience without the concern of worrying others. They also just need to say the things they are feeling—the hard things. This is a safe place for them to work through their emotions.

By creating friends and a space to always connect, through our closed Facebook page, whenever these feelings come up, they can share them. Letting emotions out can be healing during this process.

Appreciation

> *I love group today, thank you Sarah! Appreciate you so much when I come to talk it just makes me feel better.*
> *Thank you for everything and helping me come this far.*
> *I have really benefited. Thank you.*
> *I just wanted to say thank you 4 everything. I appreciate you a lot.*
> *Thank you for your help and support. I really appreciate it.*
> *Because I miss Sarah.*
> *Thank you this was very helpful.*

To this day, I am amazed at how these young adults trust me. They know I deeply care about their well-being. Being a professional social worker and dedicating my career to oncology they seem to really engage and trust me. For that I am thankful. When you hear positive feedback about the efforts you are putting in, you know it's working on a deep level of intervention.

That being said, any professional that puts in the necessary time and effort, can be trusted. Ones who are providing this type of support to young adults will see the difference they are making. The growth that the group experiences is profound. One becomes a better clinician by engaging in this type of work.

Once these young adults begin to have some small positives in their lives, it sparks makes a continuing change for the better in their lives. They then start to see more appreciation for others in their lives and they are able to communicate this to others. The benefit of small gratitude can elevate their lives and it begins in this group.

Safe Place

> *Socializing, advise, Comradery*
> *More socializing people I can relate to.*
> *Safe place to talk.*
> *Today was small group. Good talk. Scared a bit for any larger group meet ups because I am not good in groups. Main reason for coming today.*

The fact that these young adults take a chance to join a group is a big step. Creating a safe place to discuss hard things in life is valuable after going through cancer. This is so important in their process to living after cancer. Once they have a safe place to discuss their cancer experiences, they can keep coming back to that safe place to work through their issues. It opens time and space in other aspects of their life so they can be in the moment.

Feel Good

I feel good and things are going well.

Love coming to group.

What I got out of group was a well needed distraction. It was fun hanging out with everyone from group.

Because I was looking forward to this and I enjoy coming to group!!

I feel a lot better now that I spoke to my group friends.

I came today to keep the experience going. I've enjoyed coming to the last two meetings.

I came to keep my streak of consecutive attended group meetings.

I got some fun from group and sharing stories with others.

Perspective, socializing, entertainment.

Needed a distraction to get my mind off things.

Really good and revive.

I feel better overall and excited for next group.

Thanks for the motivation to keep improving and new ways to relieve stress.

Thank you for inviting me, I had an amazing time, this experience truly helped me and I plan on coming as much as I can!

You and awesome support group leaser. You always help me every time I come.

Thank you for everything.

Take a minute the recognize the good things you do for your clients and treat yourself from time to time.

Your meaning in life and is to be who you were meant to be and everyone who is in contact with your loves you for it.

As you read the information from these pre and post evaluations you understand the impact of this group in their lives. It also gives insight to how structure relevant themes for the groups you have.

Feeling welcome in a safe space with peers that have gone through cancer is the key to a successful group. Balancing the tough discussions with some happier bonding sessions is vital to the success. This group has always started with a casual meal together and I think that is worth the effort. Casual talk gets these young adults comfortable while enhancing their social skills. It comforts and welcomes some at the meal before the group sessions.

Coordinating with the young adults to simply participate in fun events together is an important element of a successful group. Some of the most significant growth has happened at casual event (i.e., a paint night, for example).

Recognizing the flow of the group and really incorporating the positive experiences is a great way to keep the members engaged and eager to keep participating in the group.

Post-Traumatic Growth

> *I have been thinking that even once I move out of state, eventually I would like to find a way to mentor/support AYA patients/survivors in the future.*
> *Group was fun I enjoyed the new people I met and their stories.*
> *I came tonight to see everyone before the new year.*
> *Thank you for a great end to 2019. Wishing the whole group good health.*

It amazes me that young adults are always able to focus on their peers. If someone is really struggling, then the others pull together to provide support. This deep need to give back is prevalent in each session. They respect others by listening and then suggesting or sharing similar experiences.

When they hear someone is having a hard time and didn't attend group, they reach out. There have been times where one member will contact me and ask me to reach out. Some will encourage their peers to attend group.

Another amazing thing is that these young adults have done a lot of volunteering. They are always willing to share their experiences and help within our community. I appreciate how they always want to give back within the group and beyond.

Cancer Treatment Reactions

> *I got great advice in regards to my weird seizurish reaction.*
> *Tips from other cancer survivors on life after treatment.*
> *I am here because it's good to get outside, and cancers been on my mind more since its MRI time.*

Many of the young adults have faced death due to a reaction from treatment. Many have had reactions that have set them back or caused life-threatening experiences. Most of the treatments can have severe adverse effects and when you listen to their experiences it's very traumatic. These young adults need to share these hard times since they were such a trauma in their lives. Hearing these traumatic experiences helps a clinician better understand the cancer experience.

Group Zoom Evaluation

> *I came to group because I thought it would be great to do something that gave me peace before COVID*
> *I came to group because I haven't been in around a month. I have had a lot of stuff going on and wanted advice and wanted to update everyone on everything.*

Tonight really helped me notice that I have been doing really well even with setbacks. That this infection is just a minor thing and that I can get past it.

Love tonight's zoom. Left me in peace. Thanks for your endless love and support.

Adjusting your community support group to keep connected through all the times of the world is important.

What has group given you?

It's given me a place where I can't talk to others who get it in a world where I no longer feel normal

Why do you attend group?

To find others who understand the same feelings I go through and to validate the weird emotions I have that other people my age cannot relate to.

How does group impact your life?

It makes me feel more normal, to have a community like me, and I feel better being able to talk to them

What unresolved issues did you have from cancer when coming to group?

Talking to friends who don't understand my outlook on life or even can understand where I am coming from

To give back to other young adults with cancer, what advice do you have from your experience in group?

You aren't alone, there are others that feel the way you do and have gone through similar experiences, it helps to reach out and find them.

What are some life lessons you want to share from your experience?

Life may not happen the easy you plan or want it to but you will end up where you need to be by the end of it.

What Has Group Given You?

Knowing that there are other people who have suffered from the same relatively uncommon condition of childhood cancer, and being able to interact with them, is a valuable resource because it reinforces the important notion that we are not alone. Many people lack sufficient enough understanding of what exactly being a young adult cancer survivor entails, or may sympathize without knowing the full picture.

Why Do You Attend Group?

As for why I attend group, going through cancer has left me with unfortunate health issues that render me unable to get a job or go to college, which are typically the main venues of real-life social interaction for other people. Being able to socialize is good for me and my self-improvement.

I have always been a person to plan things. Cancer doesn't let you do that. You go along the calendar that your cancer and your body's recovery time sets. For a person like me, that brings a lot of anxiety and depression. I had had anxiety and depression before chemo but oh not like this. My family orientation did not help neither. It was difficult having to put my life on hold, have so much uncertainty, while being around so much negativity. This support group gave me one of the two outlets I could use. All of the other people had already been out of chemo and on with their lives. It helped show me that you truly can have a happy healthy life after cancer. To be honest the only reason I started going to group was because my social worker severely suggested I go especially after having a chemo toxicity to Methotrexate and Cisplatin. That toxicity made me so terrified and not having the greatest support made things a million times worse. I was super scared about going to a support group mostly. It's these new people that I won't know, talking about cancer. I'm gonna hate it. But boy was I wrong. I instantly got along great with every person I met. My very first visit, I got so much advice on coping skills and ways other people help calm themselves when they feel things are out of control. The support I needed to positively help me get through this hardship in my life was here. The people would help me work through the uncertainty feelings I would experience. I have had a very hard time learning to adapt to my body after cancer. Having a femur resection and total knee replacement was the hardest part. I had to relearn to walk. I was severely mean and unempathetic to myself. The recovery process was, in my opinion, way to slow. I just wanted to get back to the way I was before cancer. I wanted that so desperately that after chemo, I rushed back to work and would work a lot and for long hours. I knew my body couldn't handle it but I just wanted to be like before. Well alone chemo does things that change your body. It took me a year after being cancer free, needing another knee replacement surgery because of fluid building up around my prosthesis to realize taking it easy is okay. Sleeping because you're exhausted is okay. You don't have to constantly be on the go to make life good. If it weren't for this support group, I don't think I would've ever realized that listening to my body is EXTREMELY important. Because of that, I can start after this new knee surgery with an open mind and ears ready to go based off what my body needs; not focusing on what I want.

Group has impacted my life for the better, gave me a sense of support that is difficult to find after navigating life after cancer. It has allowed me to learn about coping mechanisms and how to practice self-care. It has allowed me to build friendships and connect with other in the cancer community. Group inspires, supports and builds a positive self-identity after undergoing cancer.

Please note that two of the current members have been inspired by completing the impact of the group form. They stated in the group on 8/27/20 that they are going to write a book about their cancer experience.

Index

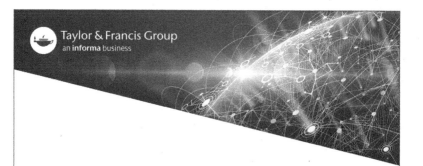